I0799996

IMAGES
of America

TOLEDO STATE HOSPITAL

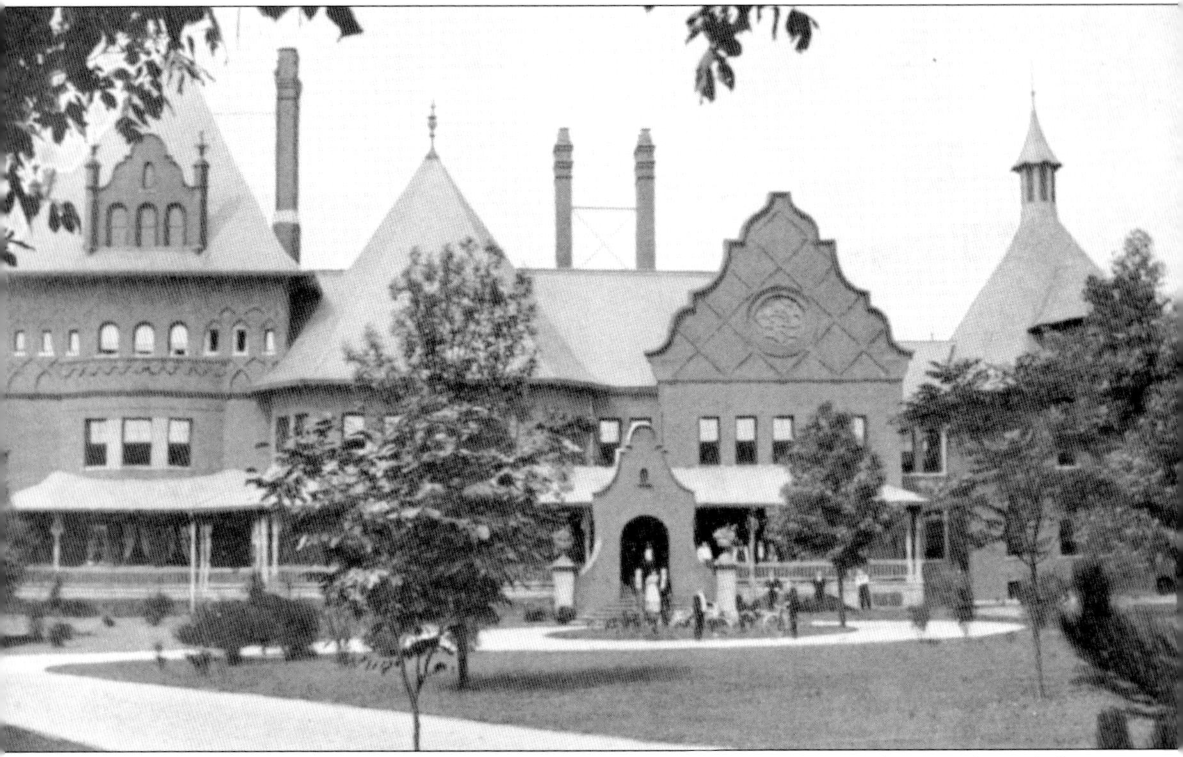

The Men's Hospital was completed in 1899. The Men's Strong Ward was enlarged that year also and was incorporated into the structure of the new hospital building. The addition of the new men's hospital, along with the larger strong ward, increased the hospital's capacity to 1,600. Two men stand beside bicycles in front of the arch in this photograph. (Northwest Ohio Psychiatric Hospital.)

ON THE COVER: Patients who were well enough to do so were free to walk from their cottages to the dining halls at mealtime. These women and their attendants pause in front of the women's cottages, perhaps returning from the dining hall, chapel, or just a walk in the fresh air and sunshine around 1888. (Local History and Genealogy Department of the Toledo Lucas County Public Library.)

IMAGES
of America

TOLEDO STATE HOSPITAL

Kimberly Brownlee

ARCADIA
PUBLISHING

ISBN 978-1-4671-0488-3

Published by Arcadia Publishing
Charleston, South Carolina

Printed in the United States of America

Library of Congress Control Number: 2019954265

For all general information, please contact Arcadia Publishing:
Telephone 843-853-2070
Fax 843-853-0044
E-mail sales@arcadiapublishing.com
For customer service and orders:
Toll-Free 1-888-313-2665

Visit us on the Internet at www.arcadiapublishing.com

This book is dedicated to those who suffer from mental illness and to those who love them. May you find peace.

Contents

ACKNOWLEDGMENTS

My greatest thanks go to my husband, Doug Brownlee, for his unwavering support and encouragement while I worked my way through this project. He is my biggest fan, and I am grateful to have him by my side.

I owe many thanks to Laura Voelz and the professional staff of the Local History and Genealogy Department of the Toledo Lucas County Public Library for their help locating and scanning hundreds of images and, in general, going above and beyond the call of duty to help me.

To Brett Johnson, director, Northwest Ohio Psychiatric Hospital, I extend my deep gratitude for allowing me unlimited access to the historical materials and images collected in the archives room at the hospital and permission to reproduce them for this book.

I am indebted to Jane Graham Weber, chair of the Toledo State Hospital Cemetery Reclamation Project and hospital retiree. Her enthusiasm, knowledge, experience, kindness, and generosity were invaluable to me in all aspects of this project.

To Arjun Sabharwal, digital initiatives archivist at Ward M. Canaday Center for Special Collections, University of Toledo Libraries, and friend, thank you for digging into the Canaday Center's collections for those elusive photographs not available elsewhere.

My thanks to Sharon Yaros, retired hospital employee, collector, and friend, for her steadfast and perpetual willingness to share her research and knowledge and to help guide me to information.

To my friends on the cemetery committee, I wish to express my gratitude for having faith in me and for cheering me on throughout the research and writing process.

Finally, thanks to my family for their constant support, encouragement, and confidence.

Without the generous help of all these individuals, this book would not have been possible.

Unless otherwise noted, the images in this volume appear courtesy of the Local History and Genealogy Department, Toledo-Lucas Count Public Library (TLCPL), the Northwest Ohio Psychiatric Hospital (NOPH), and the Ward M. Canaday Center for Special Collections, University of Toledo Libraries (CC).

INTRODUCTION

Throughout history, society's mentally ill, disabled, and otherwise unfortunate were hidden away, locked in homes, attics, or jails when they became a danger to themselves or others or left to wander the streets and make their way as best they could. Responsibility for their care was left to their families, churches, and communities. Those eventually admitted to asylums did not fare much better. In inhumane conditions, physical restraints such as chains and straps were often used to control them, and treatment methods that would be considered torture today included shaking, bloodletting, and purging.

Dorothea Dix, early American social reformer, spent much of her life advocating for better treatment of the mentally ill. In the early 1840s, she began investigating their treatment in her home state of Massachusetts and later expanded her research to other states from New Hampshire to Louisiana. She found many being kept in jails and poorhouses in horrible conditions where abuse was commonplace. In her *Memorial to the Legislature of Massachusetts*, she wrote, "I proceed, gentlemen, briefly to call your attention to the present state of insane persons confined within this Commonwealth, in cages, closets, cellars, stalls, pens! Chained, naked, beaten with rods, and lashed into obedience." She implored them to "raise up the fallen, succor the desolate, restore the outcast, defend the helpless" and pushed for the construction and expansion of hospitals where the mentally ill could receive proper treatment. Because of her work, the lives of thousands were improved.

When Ohio became a state, its counties were mandated to provide for their mentally ill, infirm, and poor. The townships were authorized to provide "outdoor relief" to the needy, including money, food, fuel, and medical care. In 1838, Lucas County established a poor farm. Located at the southeast corner of Detroit and Arlington Avenues in Toledo, it sustained many of the county's poor, mentally ill, disabled, elderly, epileptics, and others who could not support themselves. Those who were mentally and physically able were required to work on the farm for the assistance they were given. They maintained the grounds, tended livestock, grew crops, and performed other tasks necessary to keep the farm in good working order. In 1861, the county built a small, one-story asylum on the property for the care of the mentally ill who were still being kept in jails and changed its name from the Poor Farm to the County Infirmary.

In 1867, the Ohio Board of State Charities was created. Its mission was to investigate the state's public charitable and correctional institutions and to put forth recommendations for necessary changes and additional provisions. In 1868, the board visited the Lucas County Infirmary and recorded in its annual report, "The insane building is of brick, small, and without the least adaptation to its use. In it the insane, epileptic and idiotic are kept indiscriminately as to age, sex, or condition." The next year, the board deemed the infirmary to be inadequate to house the growing number of mentally ill, and a new structure to replace the insane building was constructed and completed in 1871. This building was named the Northwestern Hospital for the Insane. The new three-story structure was designed to accommodate 75 to 100 patients and was in operation until 1888, when many of its patients were transferred to the newly constructed Toledo Asylum for the Insane, later renamed Toledo State Hospital.

By 1883, Ohio's existing hospitals were severely overcrowded, and it was estimated that over 1,000 of the mentally ill were still being housed in jails. The state responded by forming a commission charged with locating a site for a new asylum. The commission was made up of the governor, the attorney general, the secretary of state, the state auditor, and Gen. Roeliff Brinkerhoff, member of the board of state charities. After much study, the commission chose a site near Toledo: a 150-acre tract donated by the county and located on the southwest corner of Detroit and Arlington Avenues across the street from the Lucas County Infirmary. The tract was bordered by Swan Creek, and the land was fertile and good for farming. The City of Toledo agreed to supply water for the cost of pumping it, and the local gas company promised to supply natural gas at a reduced rate.

With the site selected, the commission moved on to the question of a physical design for the new asylum. General Brinkerhoff was a strong proponent of the detached ward, or "cottage system." This concept was based on the belief that abolishing mechanical restraints and housing the insane in cottages would promote feelings of self-worth and independence. It was also significantly less expensive to build—$700 per capita versus $1,100 per capita for the old style of asylums. Ultimately, the commission chose the cottage system for Toledo, making it the first asylum in the country to be built entirely on the cottage model.

Another sphere of thought regarding care for the mentally ill that emerged in the 19th century was "moral treatment of the insane." This approach called for abolishing physical restraints and treating the ill with kindness and sympathy. It was believed that the stresses of daily life caused a person to become ill, and that to place the person into an environment where they were given fresh air, nutritious food, recreation, productive work, freedom to move around, and a calming atmosphere away from those stresses would help restore the mind to health. Prominent Toledo architect Edward O. Fallis and J.W. Yost of Columbus designed the buildings with the express intent of creating a home-like environment and eliminating any prison-like features. The use of the cottage model and the practice of the moral treatment approach combined to make the Toledo State Hospital revolutionary in its early years.

The hospital opened in 1888, with Dr. Henry A. Tobey as superintendent, and the first patients were transfers from other state facilities. Over the years, the hospital grew, and treatment methods evolved. Overpopulation was a chronic problem from the beginning, and during the 1950s, the patient population peaked at just over 3,000. However, with the development of new psychotropic drugs and the availability of mental health-care services in the community, the population finally began a slow but steady decline.

By this time, the hospital's buildings had deteriorated because of age and neglect, and as they were emptied, they were razed. A new state-supported facility, the Northwest Ohio Psychiatric Hospital, now operates on the site and provides adult inpatient psychiatric care.

Today, very few traces of the once beautiful buildings and grounds remain—only a few visible remnants and two cemeteries containing the graves of nearly 2,000 former patients whose bodies were not claimed by family or friends. The University of Toledo now owns most of the former State Hospital property and is developing it into a research and technology corridor.

One

1838–1888

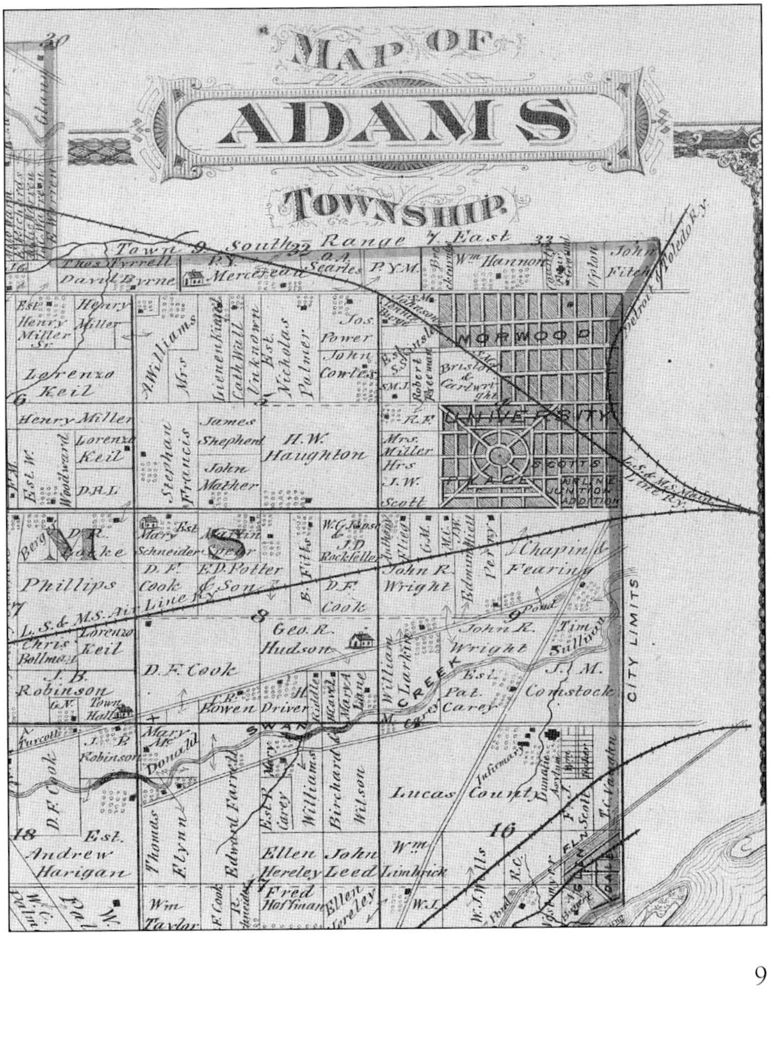

The Lucas County Poor Farm, and later Infirmary, was established in 1838 to provide care for the county's mentally ill, infirm, "friendless" elderly, epileptics, and others in need. There, they were given daily "alms," which included food, fuel, clothing, medicine, and other basic necessities. In exchange, if physically and mentally able, they were expected to do daywork on the farm. In 1861, a small one-story asylum was built there. This image is from Durant's *Illustrated Historical Atlas*. (TLCPL.)

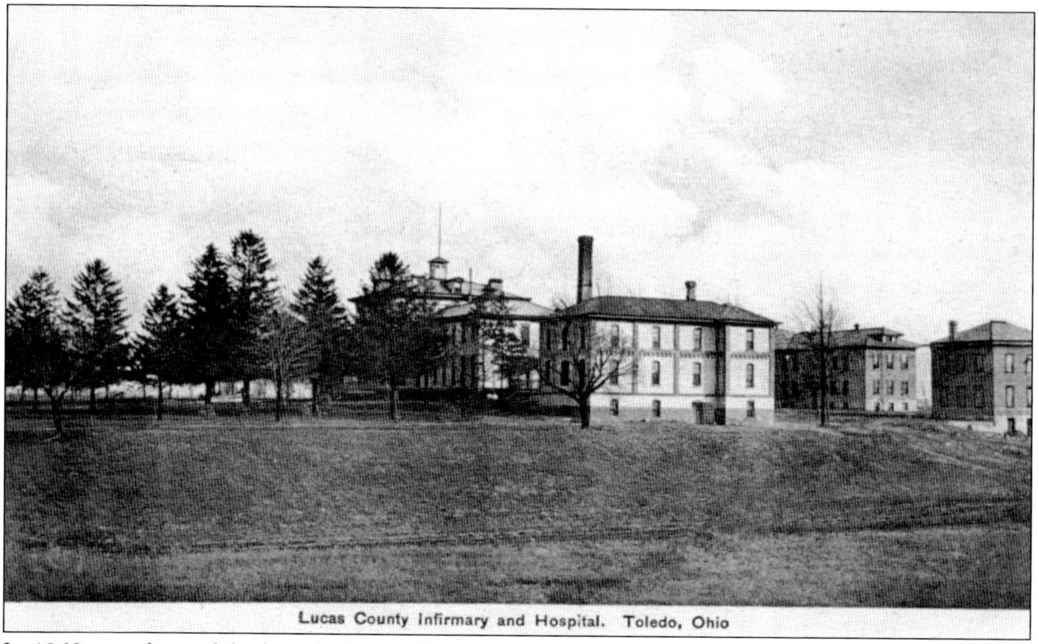

In 1868, members of the board of state charities visited the Lucas County Infirmary and reported their horror at "the general condition of the premises and the inmates." They mentioned the small asylum specifically, where "the insane, epileptic and idiotic" were kept together regardless of "age, sex or condition." The results were improvements to the existing buildings and the construction of a new asylum on the site. (NOPH.)

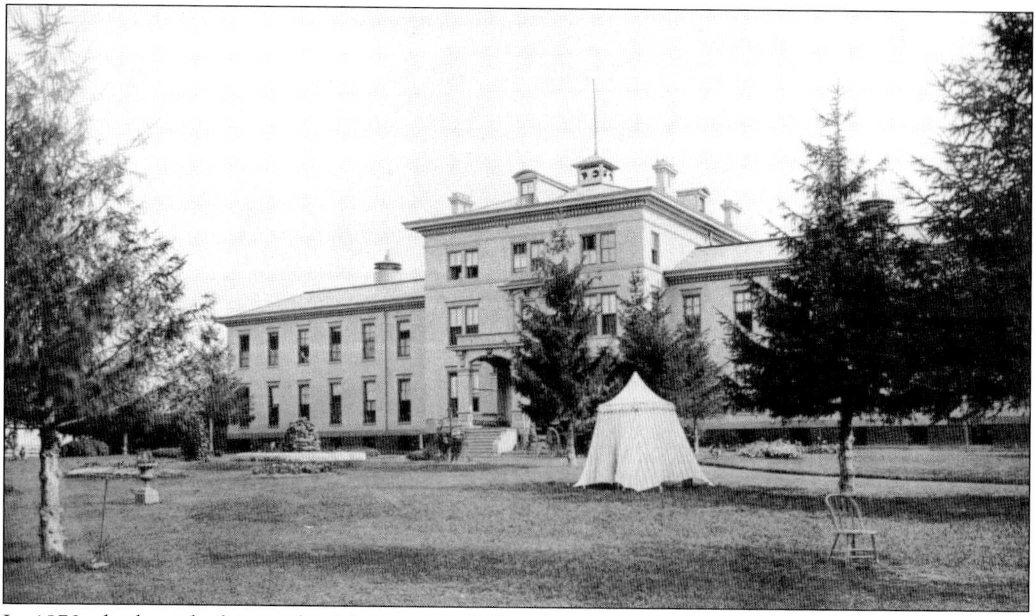

In 1870, the board of state charities reported that there were still nearly 1,200 insane being kept in infirmaries and jails in the state. Construction of the Northwestern Hospital for the Insane was completed in 1871 on the grounds of the Lucas County Infirmary. The new structure replaced the older asylum building that had become inadequate to serve the increasing number of mentally ill being housed in the county's jails. (TLCPL.)

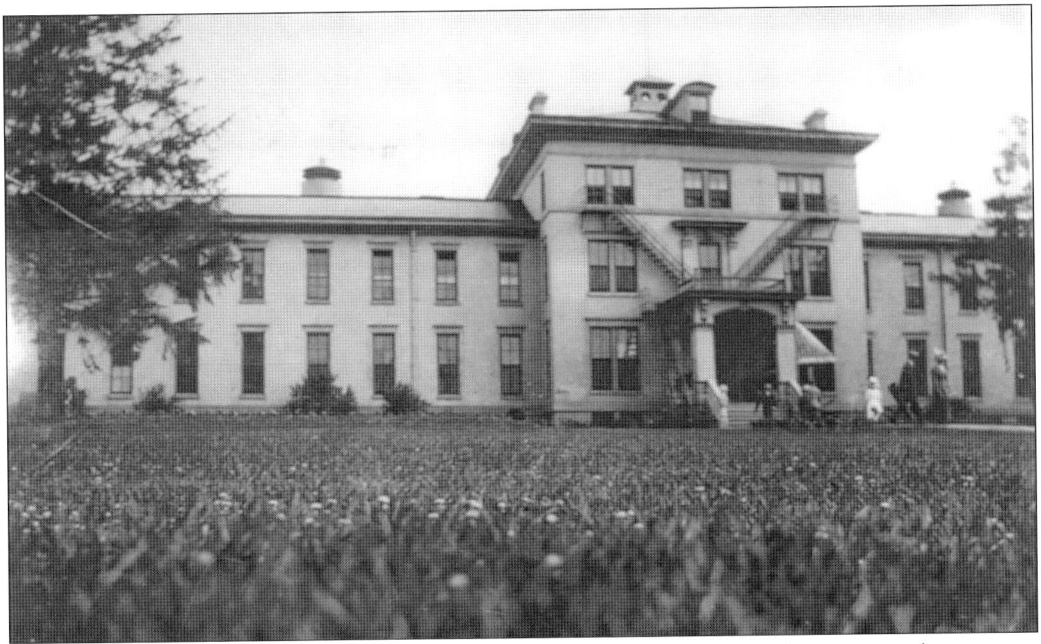

The new building was described as "an elegant and quite commodious brick structure, three stories high, and capable of accommodating [sic] from 75 to 100 patients." Although it was a county institution, it was heavily funded by the state in exchange for taking overflow patients from other state hospitals. This hospital operated until 1888, when many of its patients were transferred to the new Toledo Asylum for the Insane. (NOPH.)

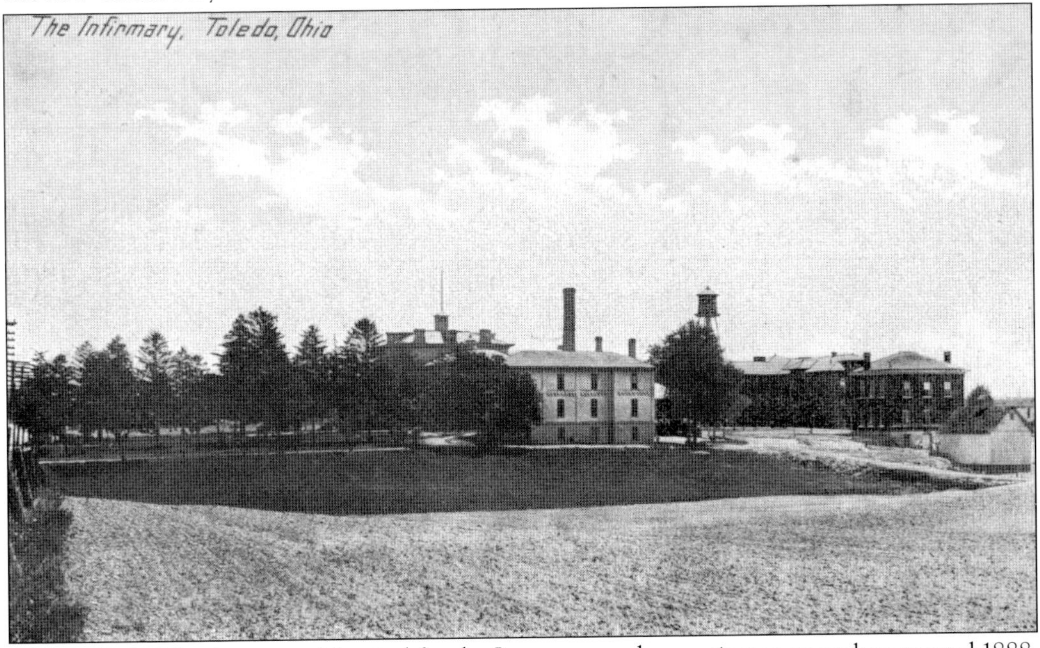

Although the Northwestern Hospital for the Insane ceased operating as an asylum around 1888, the infirmary continued its work caring for the county's sick and indigent for many years. In 1913, the infirmary's record of employees recorded that the superintendent and chief medical officer both earned $150 per month, while nurses earned only $15. (TLCPL.)

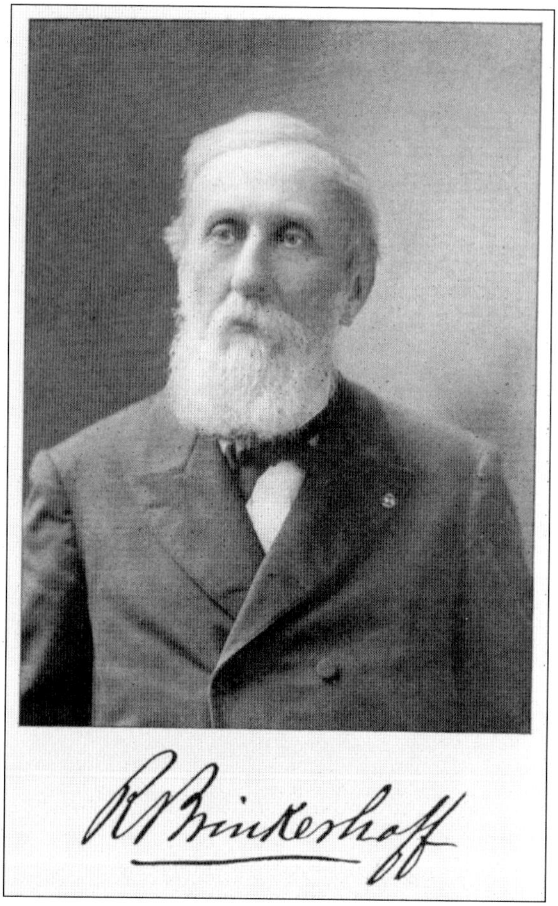

Gen. Roeliff Brinkerhoff, a member of the Ohio Board of State Charities, was appointed to the state commission tasked with locating a site in northwest Ohio for a new insane asylum. General Brinkerhoff was a strong proponent of the detached ward, or cottage system, plan for asylums. This new style was eventually chosen for the design of the Toledo State Hospital, but skeptics dubbed it "Brinkerhoff's Folly." (CC.)

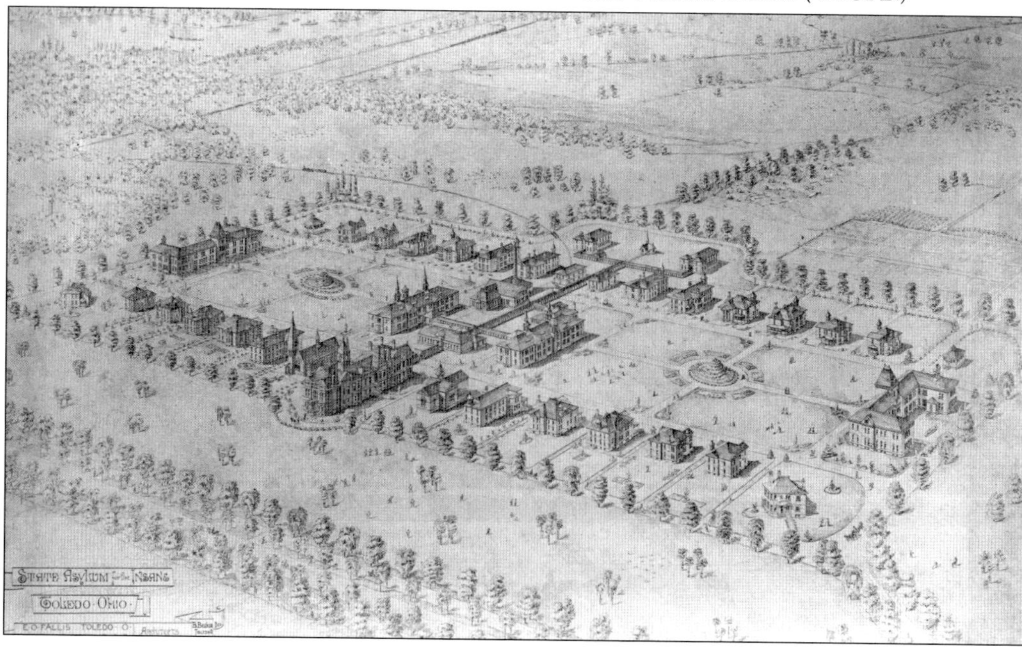

The design for the hospital was drawn by prominent Toledo architect Edward O. Fallis and architect J.W. Yost of Columbus. Fallis is known for designing other important Toledo buildings, including the Valentine Theater and the old Toledo Public Library building, built in 1890 at Madison Avenue and Ontario Street. (TLCPL.)

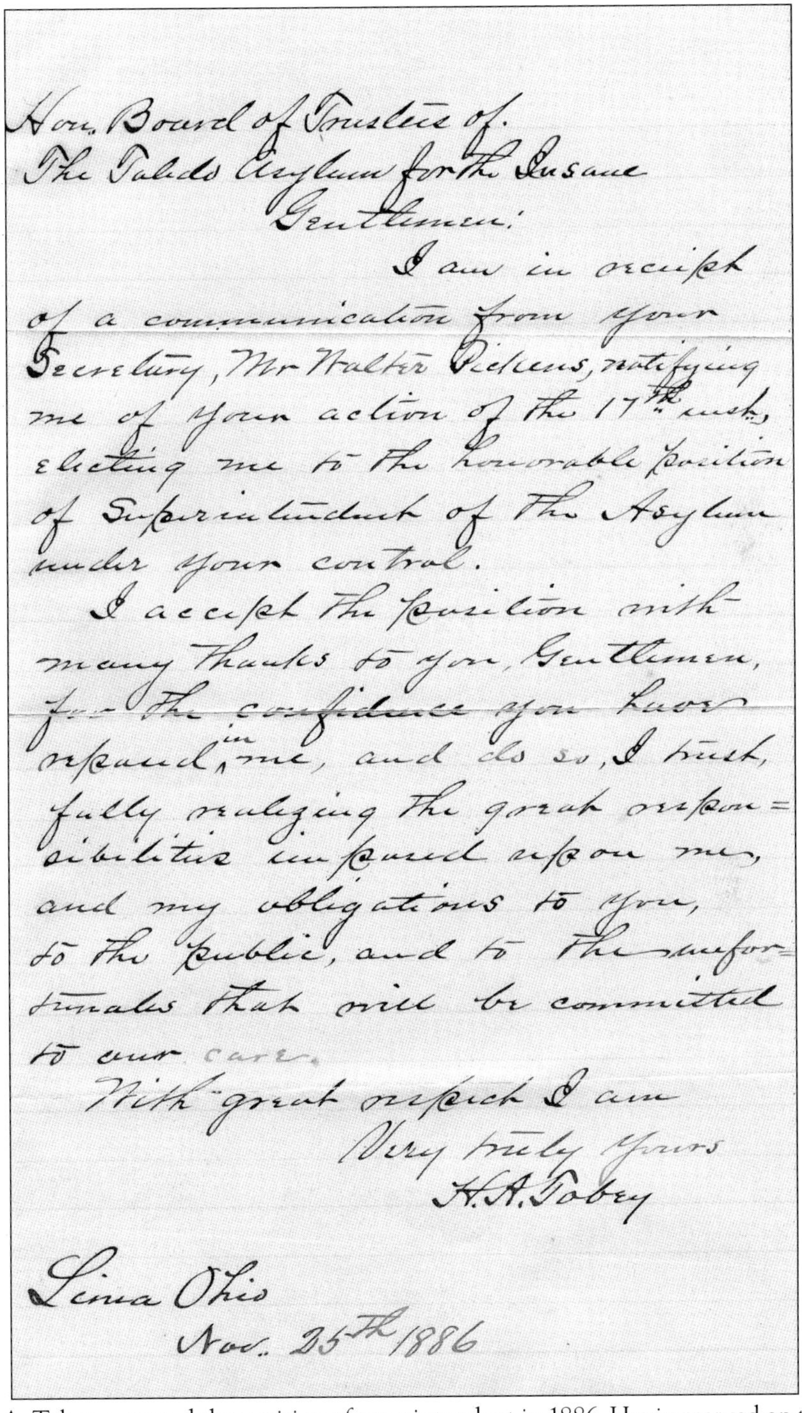

Hon. Board of Trustees of.
The Toledo Asylum for the Insane
Gentlemen:

I am in receipt of a communication from your Secretary, Mr Walter Dickens, notifying me of your action of the 17th inst., electing me to the honorable position of Superintendent of The Asylum under your control.

I accept the position with many thanks to you, Gentlemen, for the confidence you have reposed in me, and do so, I trust, fully realizing the great responsibilities imposed upon me, and my obligations to you, to the public, and to the unfortunates that will be committed to our care.

With great respect I am
Very truly yours
H. A. Tobey

Lima Ohio
Nov. 25th 1886

Dr. Henry A. Tobey accepted the position of superintendent in 1886. Having served on the medical staff at the Columbus Asylum for the Insane, and as superintendent of the Dayton Asylum for the Insane, Dr. Tobey was well prepared for the job. He was an excellent doctor, a progressive administrator, and an enthusiastic leader, and he soon brought the new and unique hospital in Toledo to international attention. (NOPH.)

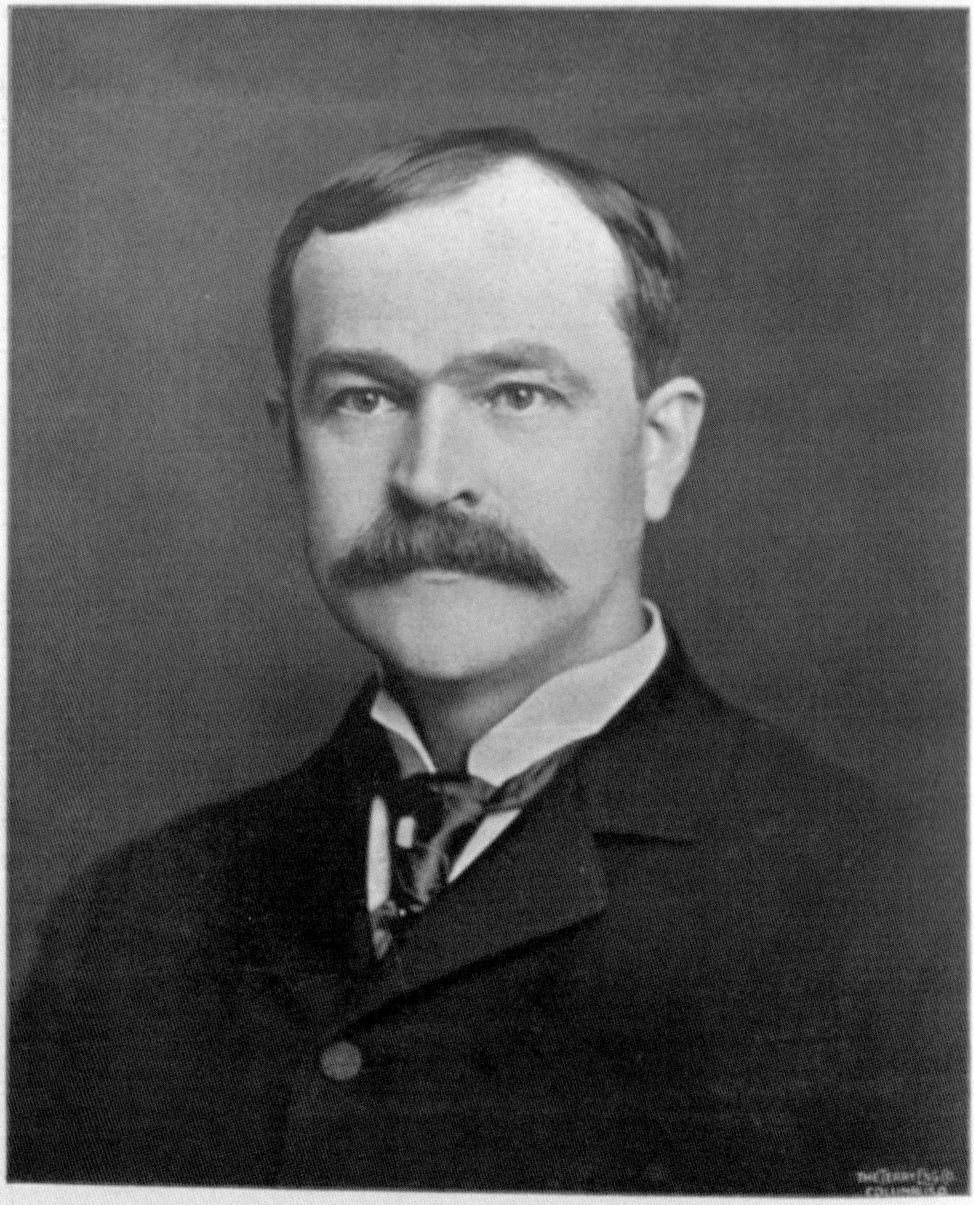

H. A. TOBEY.

Dr. Tobey was devoted to the care of the sick and afflicted in his charge, and his patients loved and respected him. His colleague Dr. Henry C. Eyman said in 1918, "If there is a place between here and Heaven where some poor soul has fallen and has sent up his cry for help, that there you will find Dr. Tobey comforting him and ministering to his needs." (TLCPL.)

Two

1888–1920

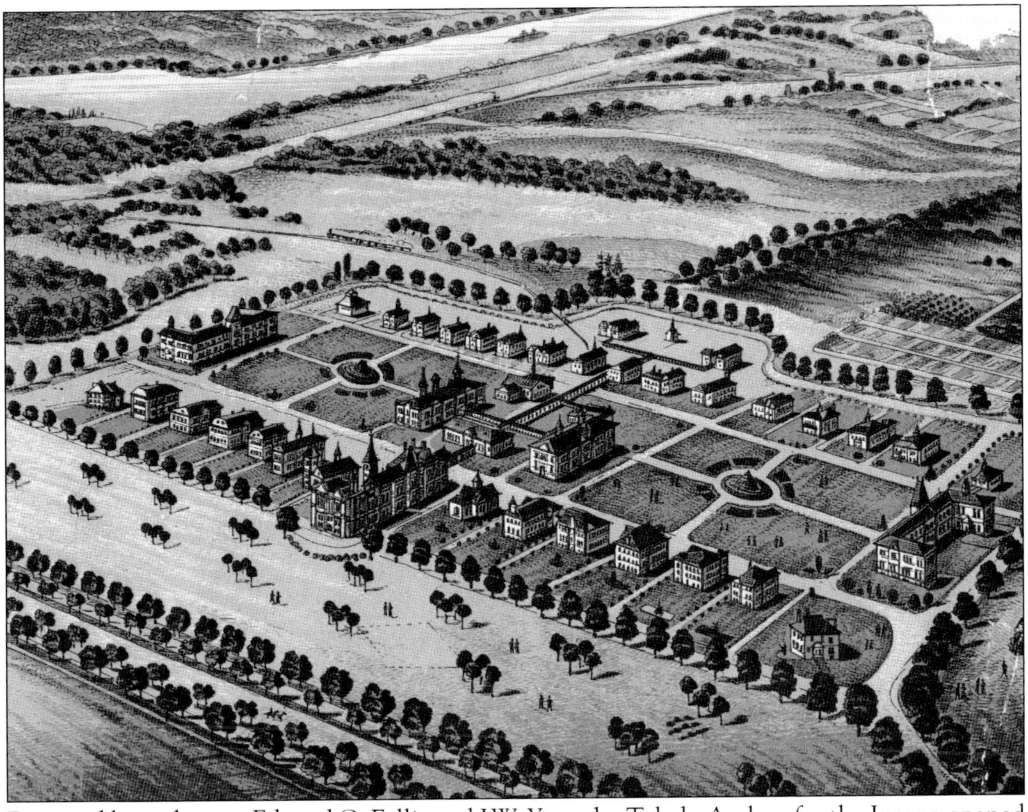

Designed by architects Edward O. Fallis and J.W. Yost, the Toledo Asylum for the Insane opened in 1888. It was situated on 150 acres of land donated by Lucas County and was constructed on the detached ward or cottage system design, a revolutionary concept at the time. Its original structures consisted of 34 buildings and could hold 1,000 patients and 200 employees. (TLCPL.)

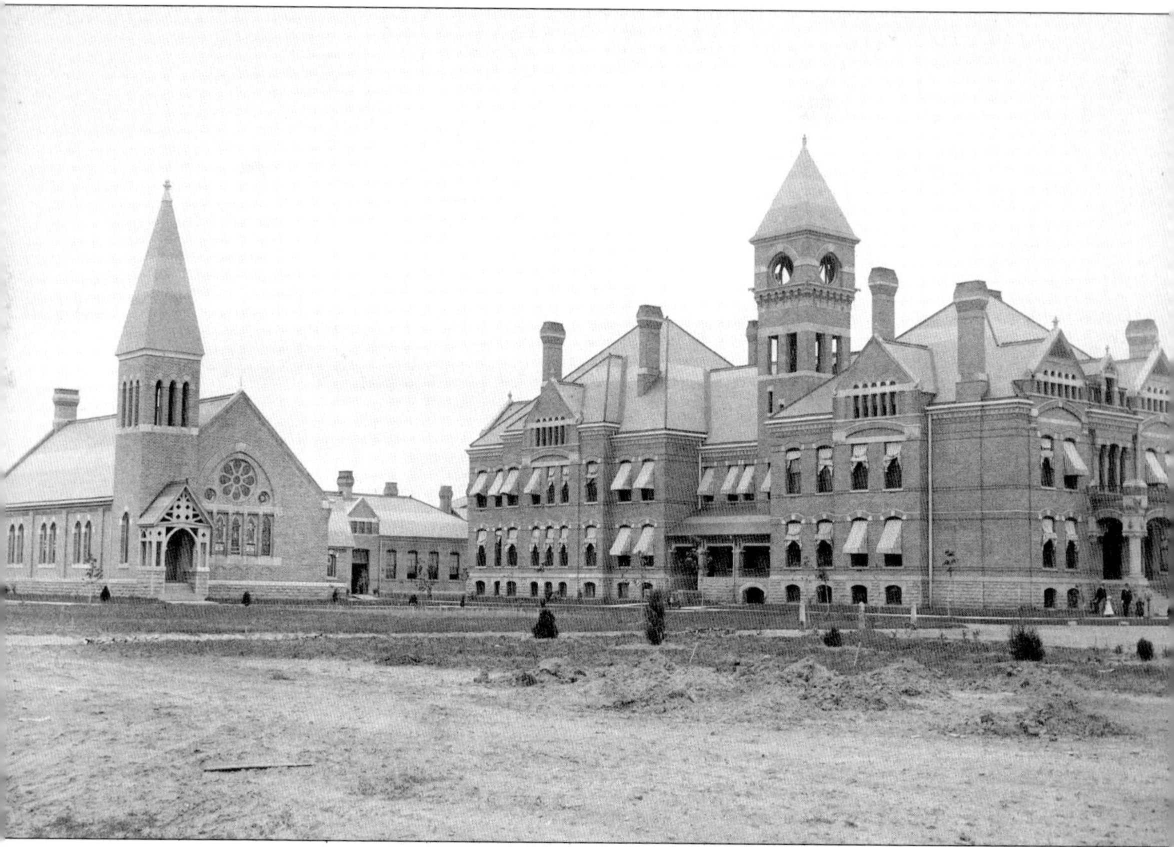

The original 34 structures of the hospital included 20 pavilions (or "cottages"), two strong wards, two infirm wards, two hospitals, an administration building, a chapel, a kitchen and bakery, a laundry, a storehouse, a boiler house, and two dining halls. Within the first 10 years, an entertainment hall and greenhouse were added, as well as several man-made lagoons. (TLCPL.)

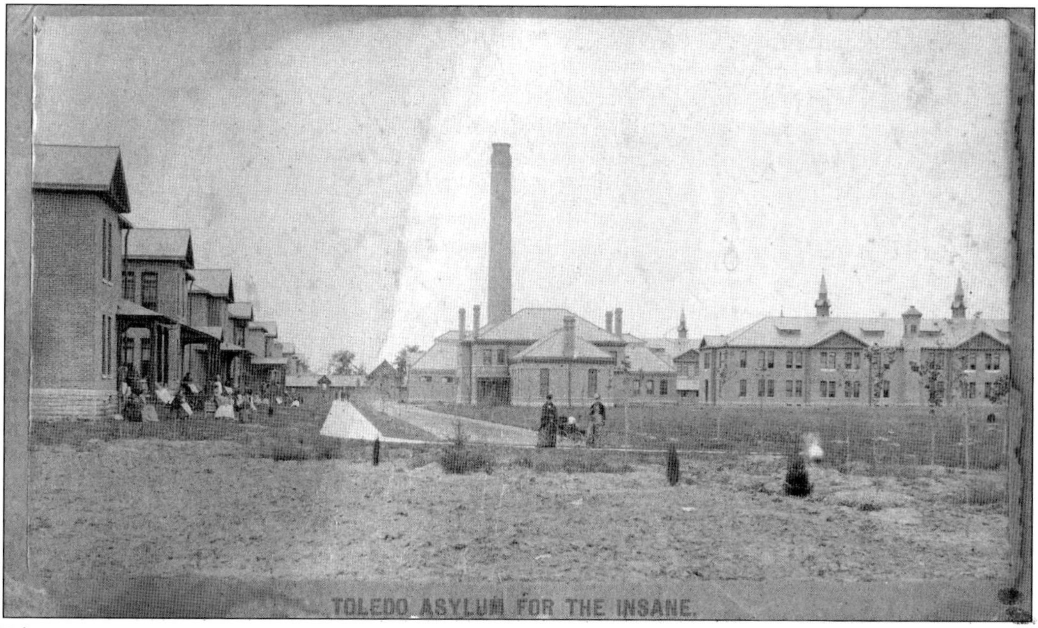

The mission statement and philosophy of the new asylum read, "To many the subject of caring for the insane is . . . a mystery. The secret of their care and keeping them contented is to have them lead as normal a life as possible, with good clean, healthy surroundings, plenty of nourishing food, and fresh air." (TLCPL.)

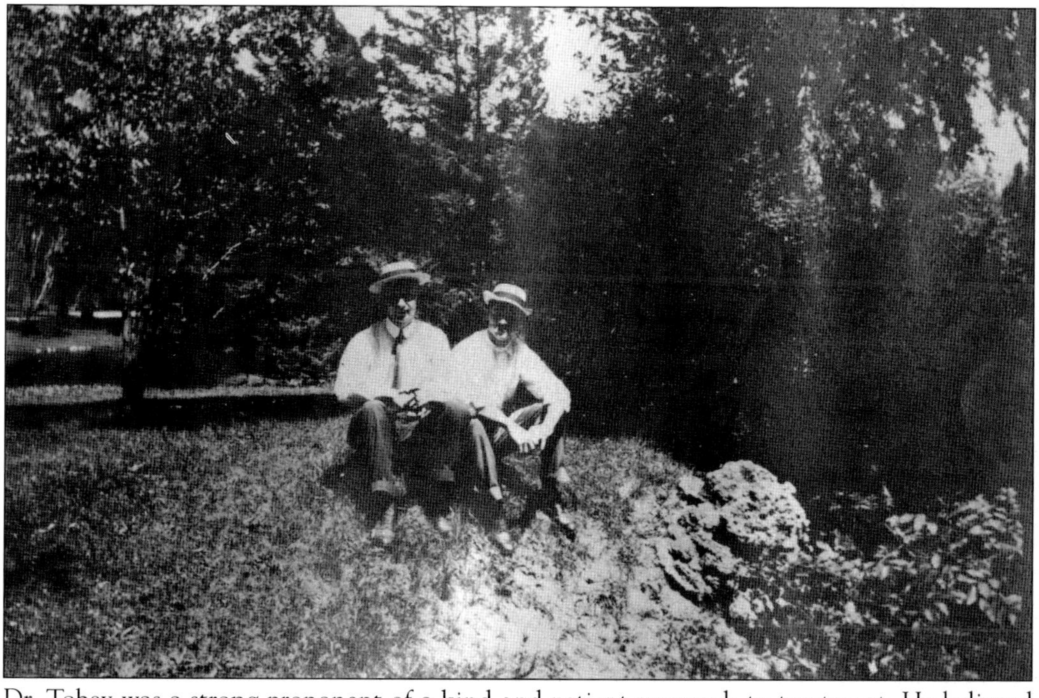

Dr. Tobey was a strong proponent of a kind and patient approach to treatment. He believed that a beautiful environment, meaningful employment, recreation, regimentation, freedom, and privileges were the best methods for restoring the mentally disturbed to health. He wished to limit the use of physical restraints to the direst of cases, if not abolish them entirely. (TLCPL.)

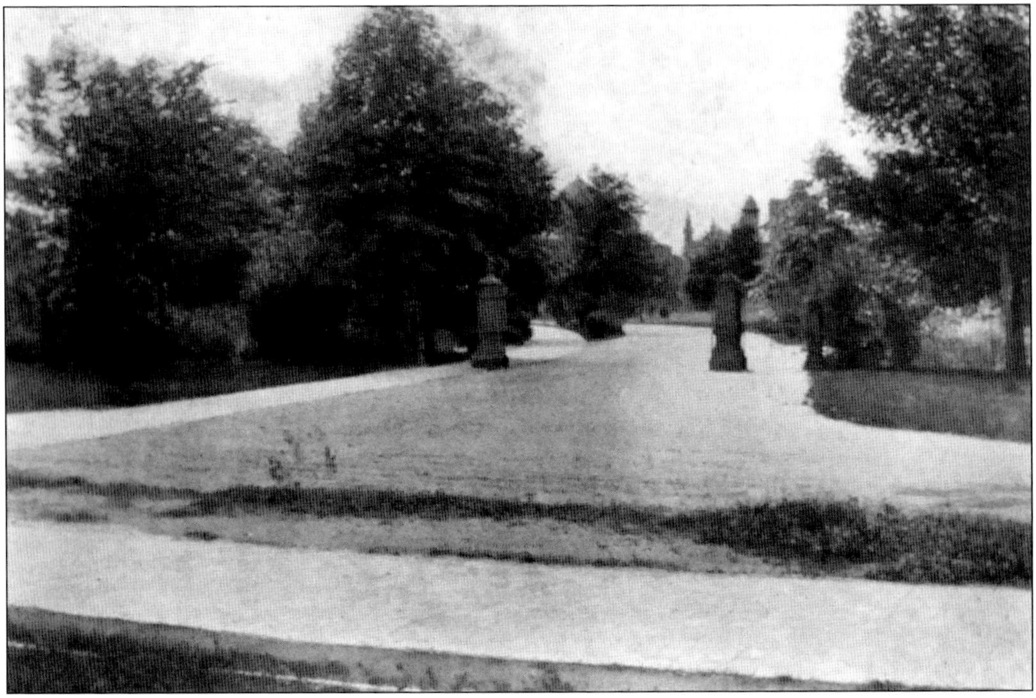

The main entrance to the hospital, pictured here around 1890, was located off Detroit Avenue in front of the Administration Building. Other entrances were located off Arlington Avenue, at the corner of Arlington and Detroit Avenues, and farther west of the main entrance off Detroit Avenue near the south lake. (NOPH.)

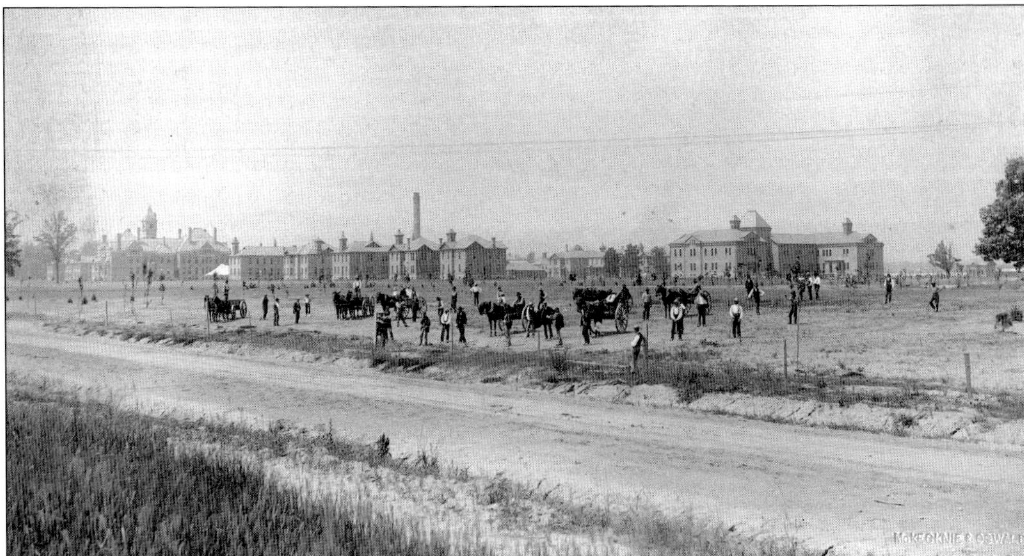

Men with horses and wagons work the grounds of the new hospital along Detroit Avenue around 1888. Male patients did much of the landscaping work on the grounds, planting flowers and trees, building the drives, and excavating the six lagoons on the property. Productive work, even menial, was an important component of the moral treatment of the insane and helped patients regain a sense of self-worth. (TLCPL.)

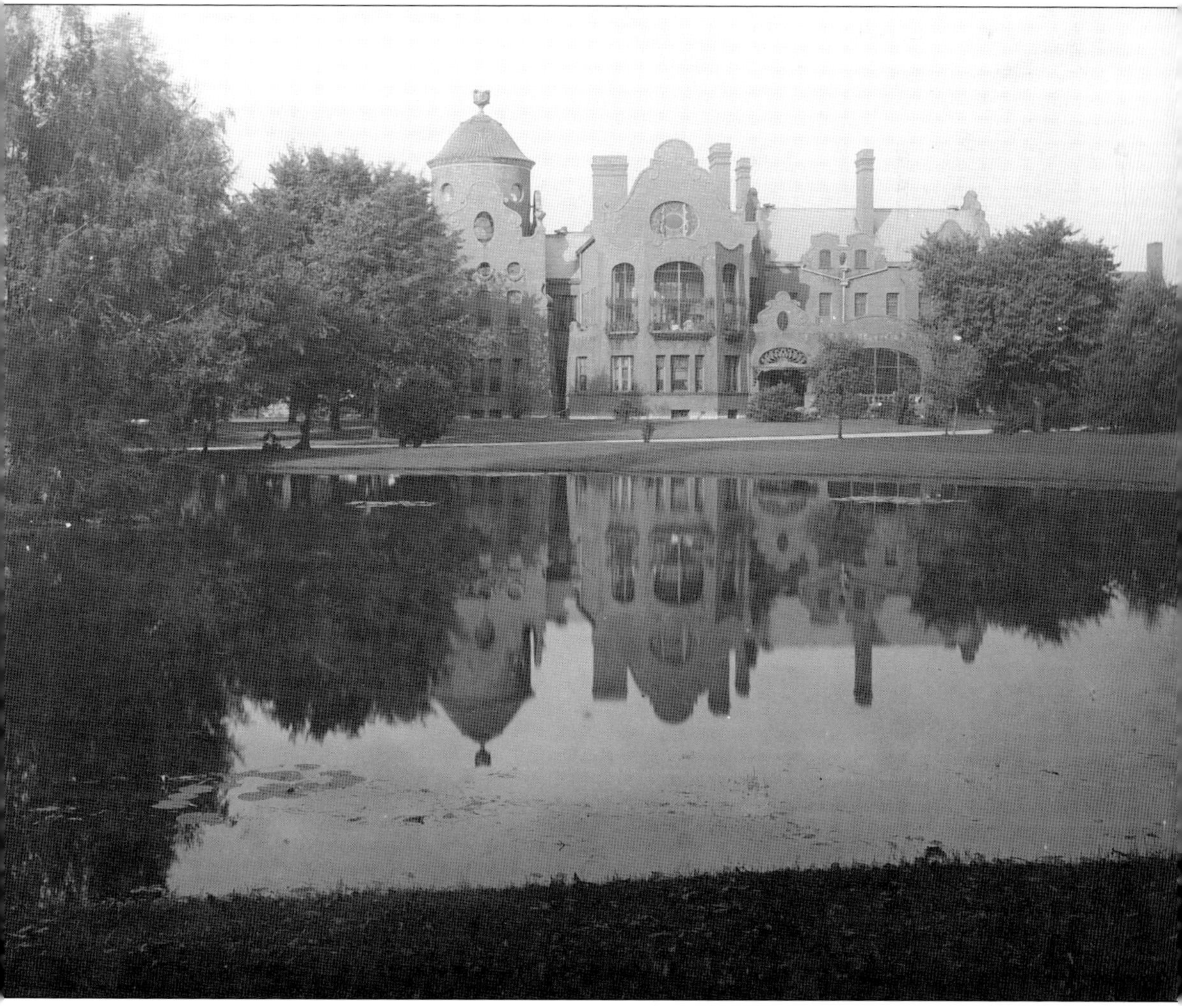

One of six lagoons on the grounds excavated by patients, this one was the largest and was known as the Sunken Garden. The lagoons added beauty to the grounds and were often the sites of picnics and special events, not only for patients but for the public as well. The large building in this scene was the Women's Hospital, completed in 1901. (TLCPL.)

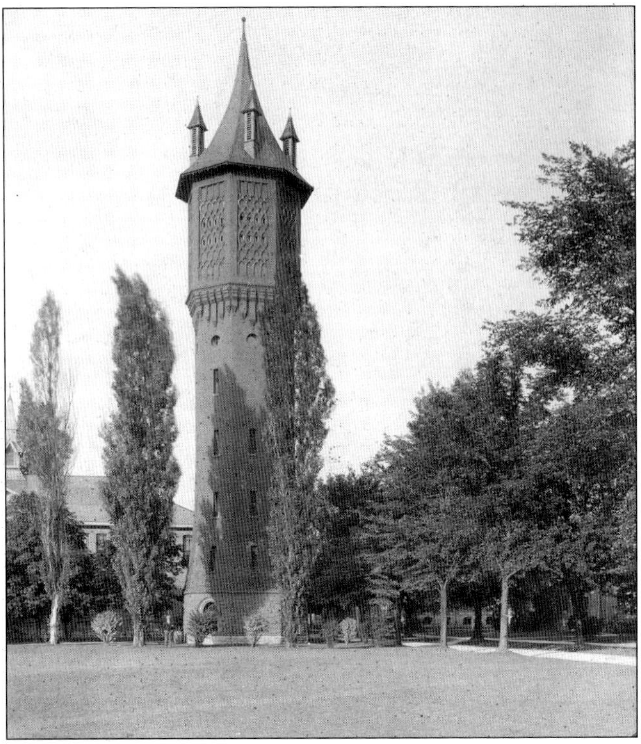

When a site for the hospital was being selected, the City of Toledo pledged to provide water for the cost of pumping it. This water tower was built in 1890 in the Gothic style of architecture and was 125 feet tall. In later years, four bedrooms were built in the upper part of the tower for night watchmen's quarters, and in 1956, it was renovated for use as a post office. (TLCPL.)

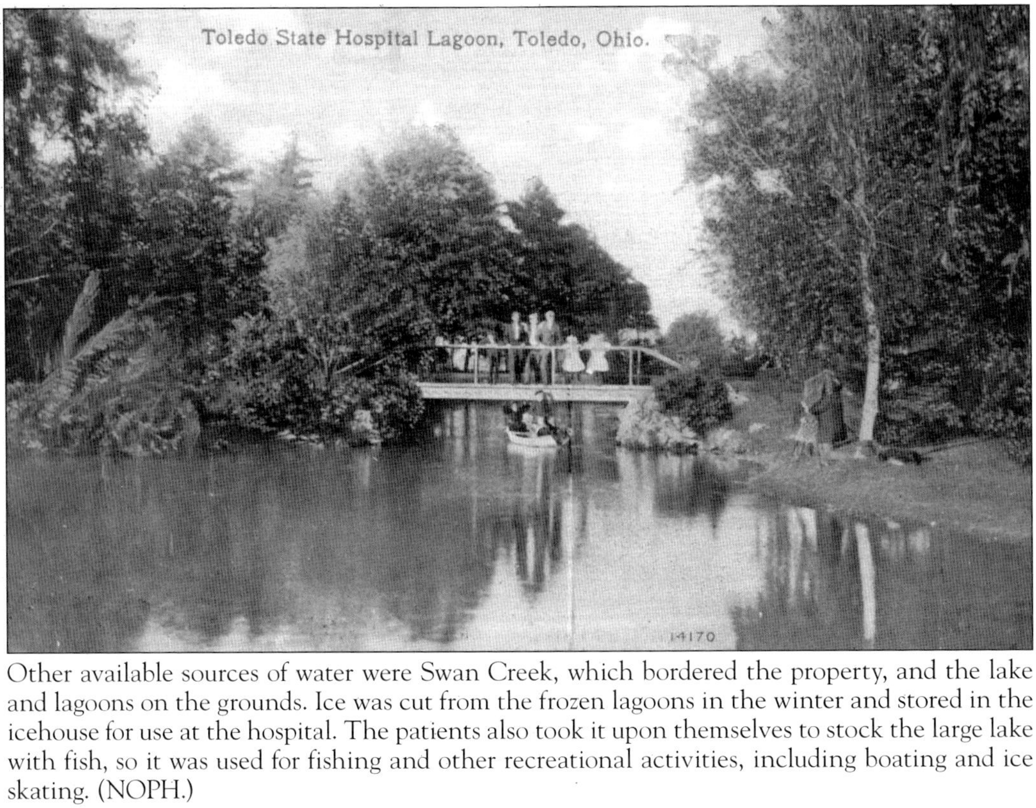

Other available sources of water were Swan Creek, which bordered the property, and the lake and lagoons on the grounds. Ice was cut from the frozen lagoons in the winter and stored in the icehouse for use at the hospital. The patients also took it upon themselves to stock the large lake with fish, so it was used for fishing and other recreational activities, including boating and ice skating. (NOPH.)

Dr. Ella Lupton was the first female physician at the hospital, serving from 1888 to 1889. She returned to her hometown of Gallipolis, Ohio, where she went into private practice and was the only female physician in that town for 55 years. Her many accomplishments included founding the Gallia County Tuberculosis and Health Association. (Gallia County Historical Society.)

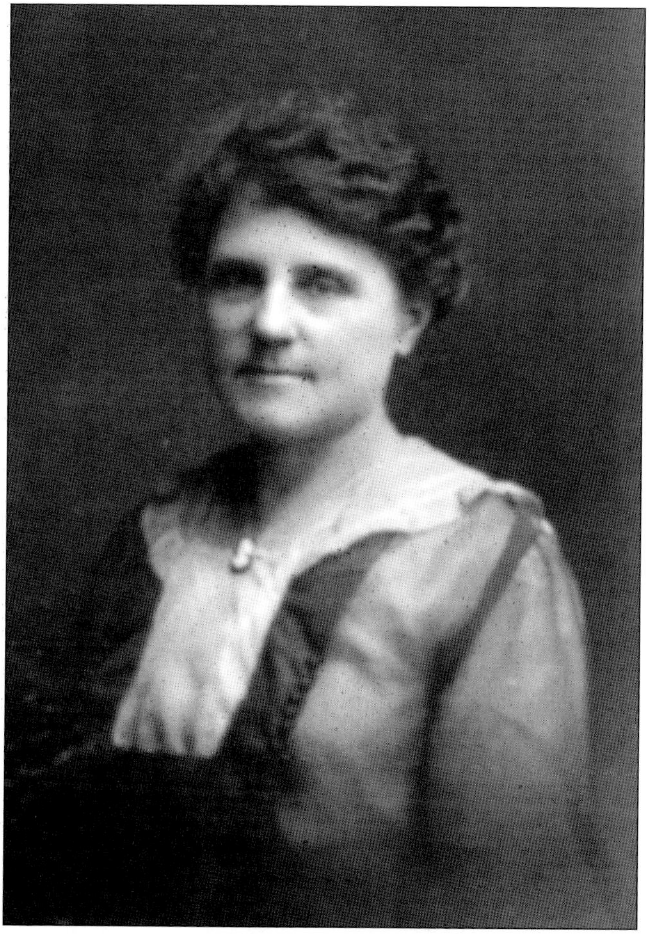

Dr. Tobey was once asked how he kept patients away from the lakes and off the boats. He replied, "We don't. There are at least 200 in the grove about the banks . . . [and] every person you see in a boat is a patient." He then quelled the visitor's concern about patient suicide, stating that "the patients have not used the water for any such purpose!" (TLCPL.)

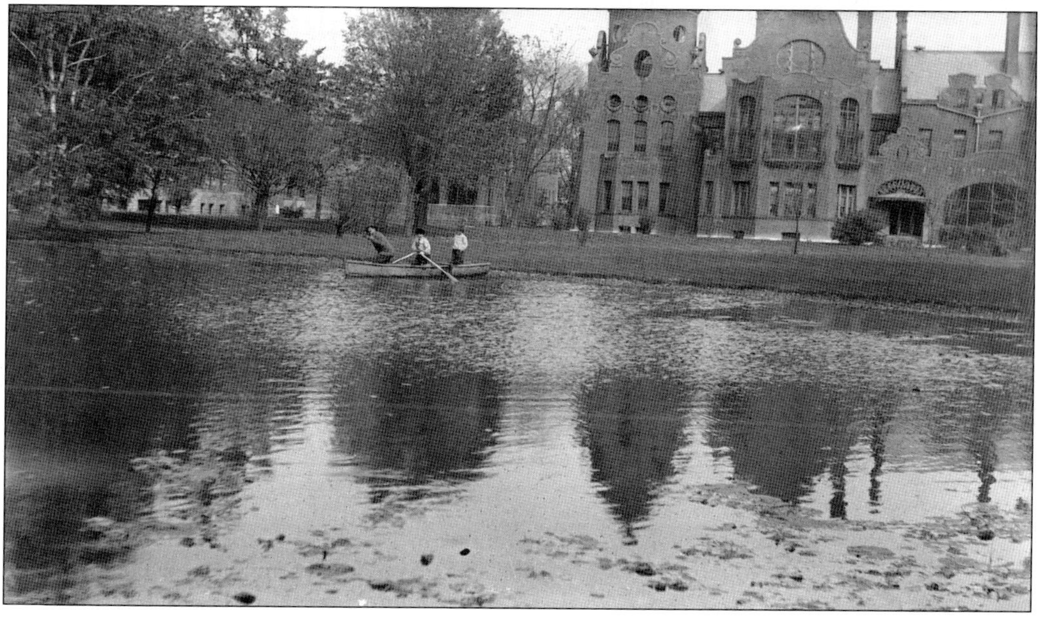

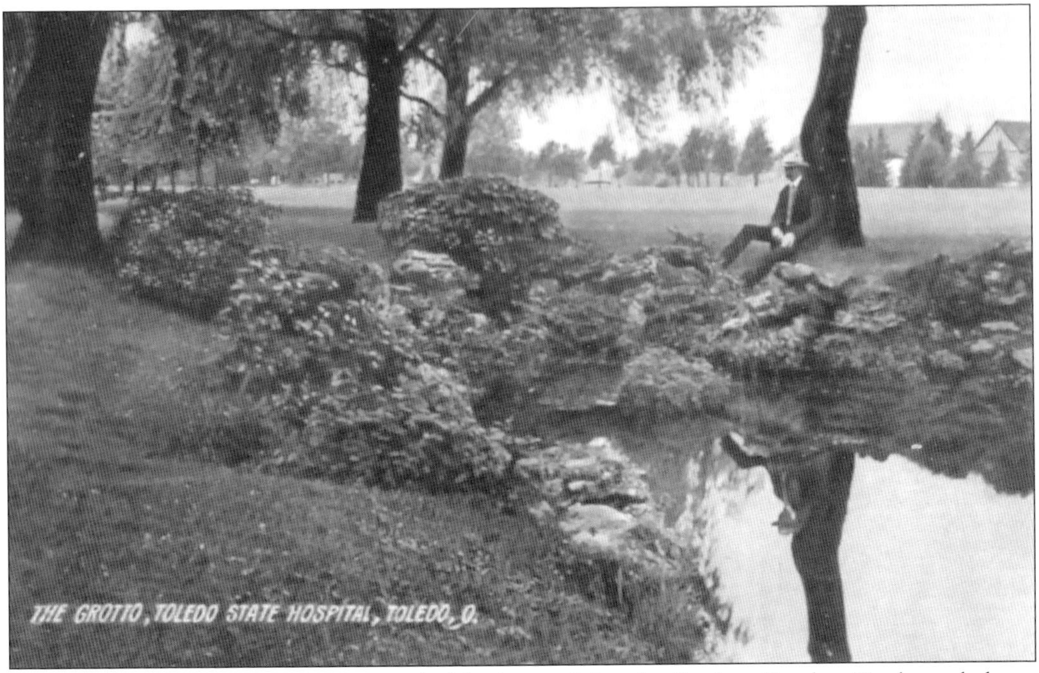

The Grotto was located at the west end of the largest lake, the Sunken Garden. Rocks and plants placed there when the lake was excavated were intended to create a peaceful atmosphere. In addition to adding to the beauty of the grounds, the lagoons provided quiet places for thought, reflection, and relaxation and thus calmed and helped heal the mind. (NOPH.)

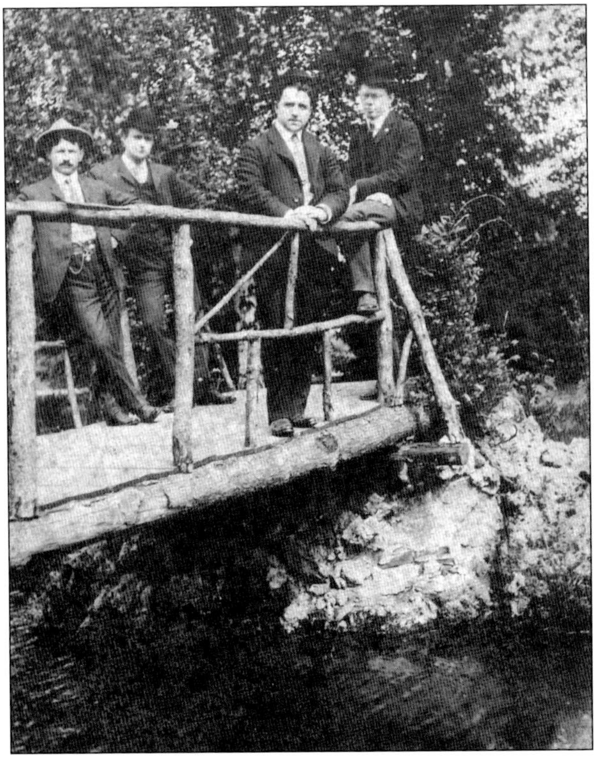

Four dapper young men pose on a footbridge across a narrow channel between two lagoons on the hospital property around 1900. The buildings and grounds of the hospital were so beautiful that they were pictured on postcards, and the park-like atmosphere was often the setting of family picnics and outings by both hospital visitors and the public. The rustic bridge was built by one of the patients. (TLCPL.)

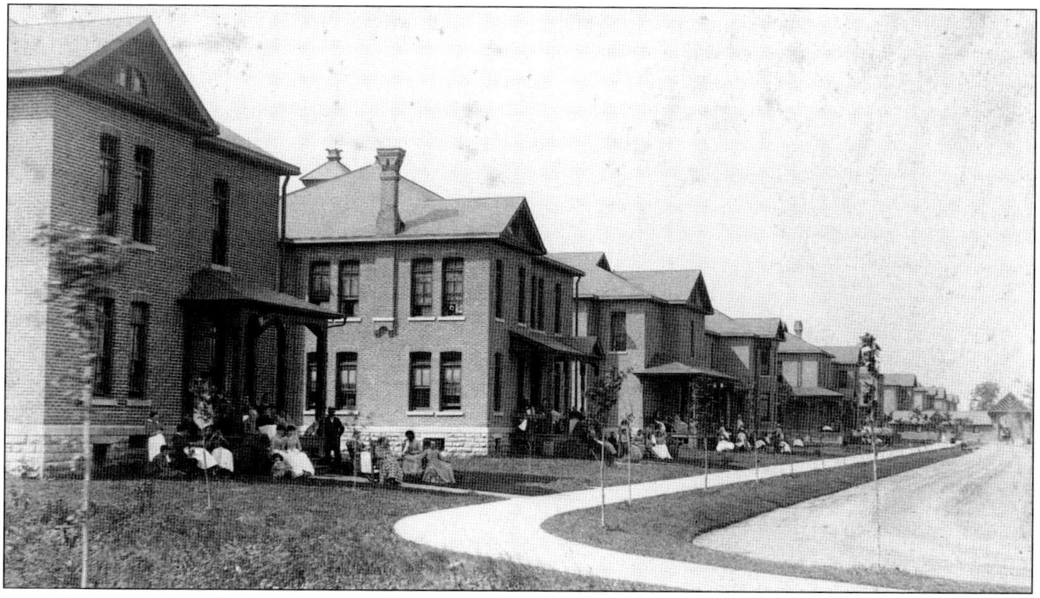

Female patients and attendants relax in the fresh air and sunshine on the lawns of women's cottages F–K around 1890. Each of the original 20 cottages was built on different designs in order to create a home-like setting and to eliminate a prison-like atmosphere so common in older asylum designs. Women's and men's cottages were located on opposite ends of the grounds. (TLCPL.)

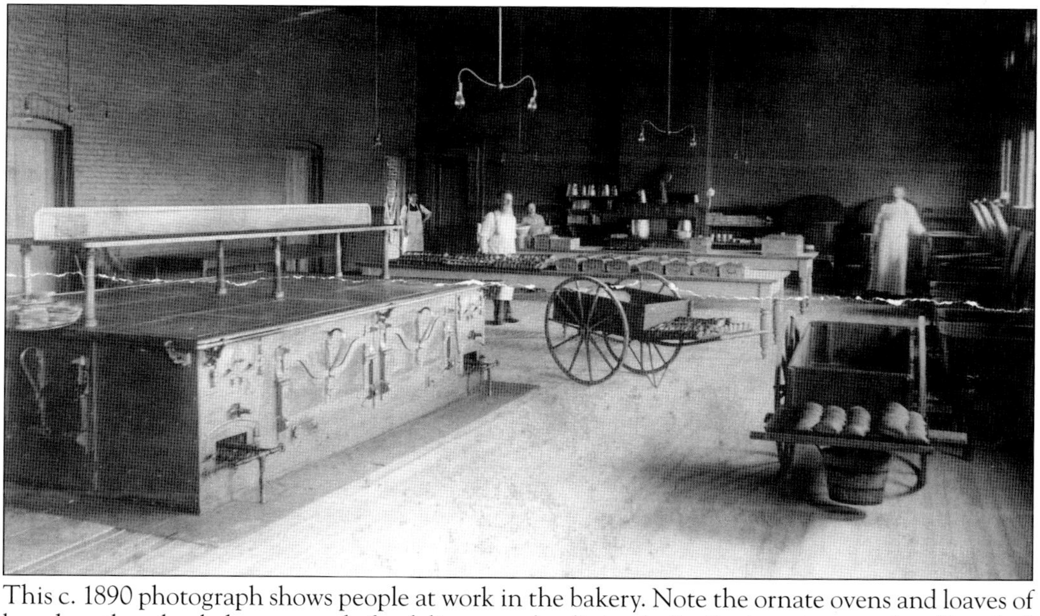

This c. 1890 photograph shows people at work in the bakery. Note the ornate ovens and loaves of bread on the wheeled carts, ready for delivery to the dining halls. Both patients and staff worked in the hospital's kitchens, peeling, cooking, baking, and cleaning. Wholesome, nourishing food was believed to help restore the ill and troubled to health. (TLCPL.)

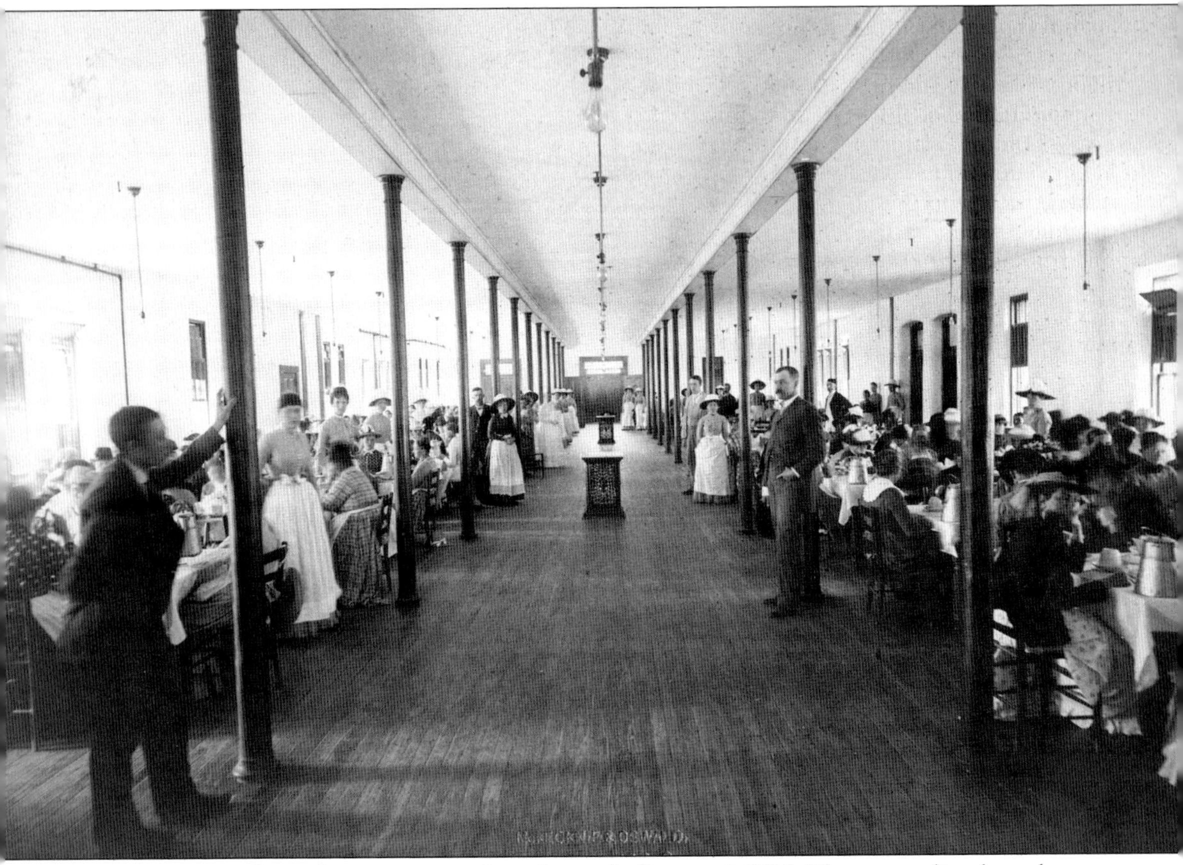

Women are shown here eating in their dining hall around 1890. Those standing by columns are attendants. One bill of fare offered such dishes as veal or mutton stew with dumplings, roast turkey with dressing and cranberry sauce, and corn beef with potatoes and fried parsnips. Patients were permitted to walk from their cottages to the dining halls at mealtime. (TLCPL.)

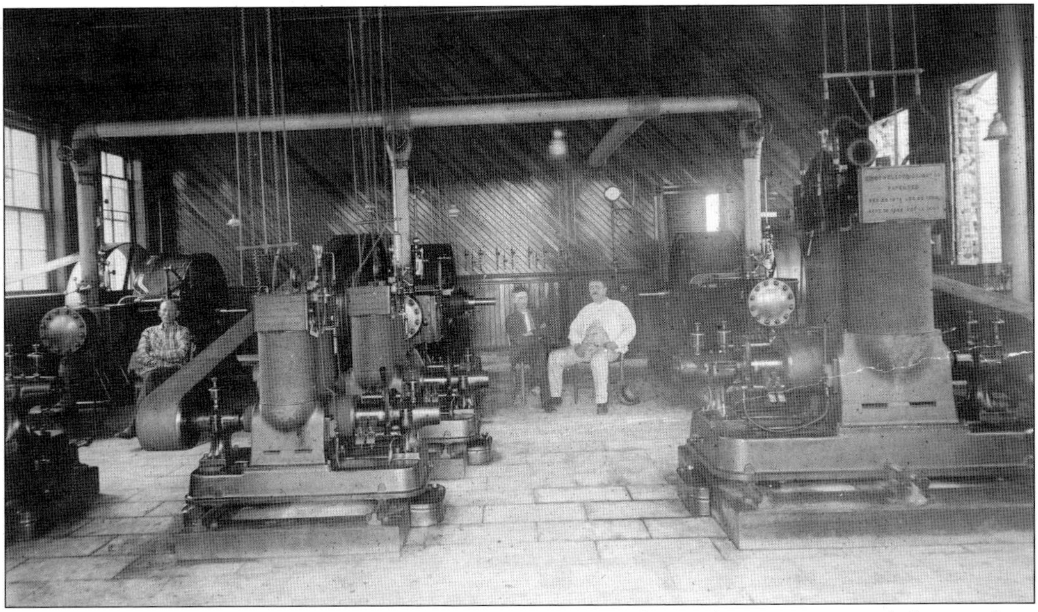

The boiler house, seen here around 1890, contained the mechanical equipment needed to produce power. The boilers used water and a heat source to create steam. The steam was then used to produce heat and to power turbines to produce electricity for the entire hospital. The men shown in this photograph are probably employees rather than patients, as boiler work was a dangerous occupation. (TLCPL.)

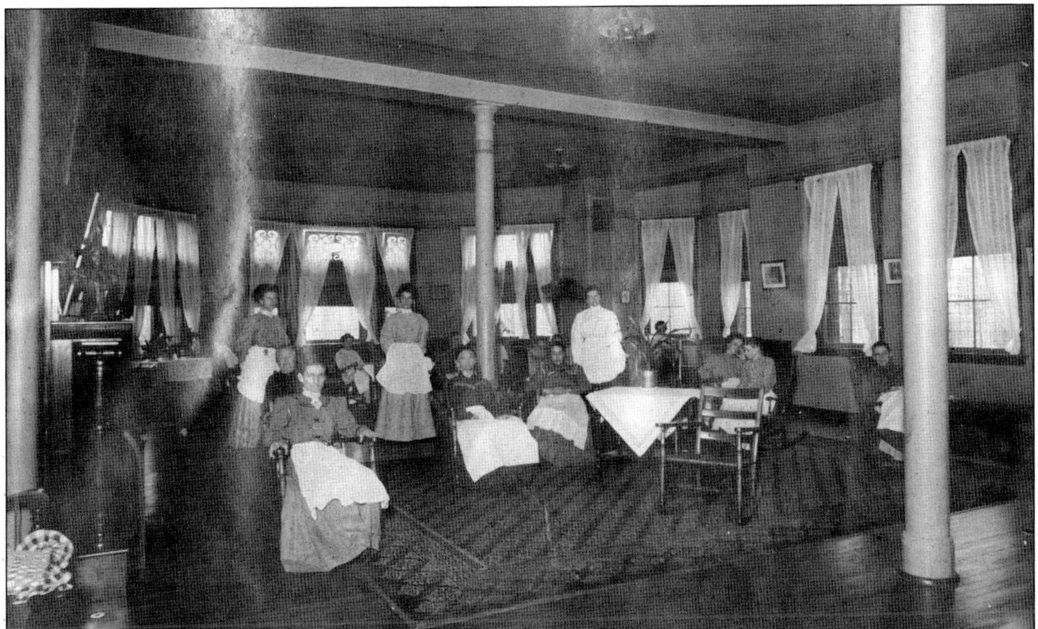

Female patients and attendants pause from their work in the parlor of one of the women's cottages. Women were busied with tasks such as sewing, weaving, rug making, and other crafts. They also performed domestic chores, worked in the kitchen, and helped with laundry. Such activities kept idle hands and minds occupied and slowly helped to restore a sense of self-worth. (TLCPL.)

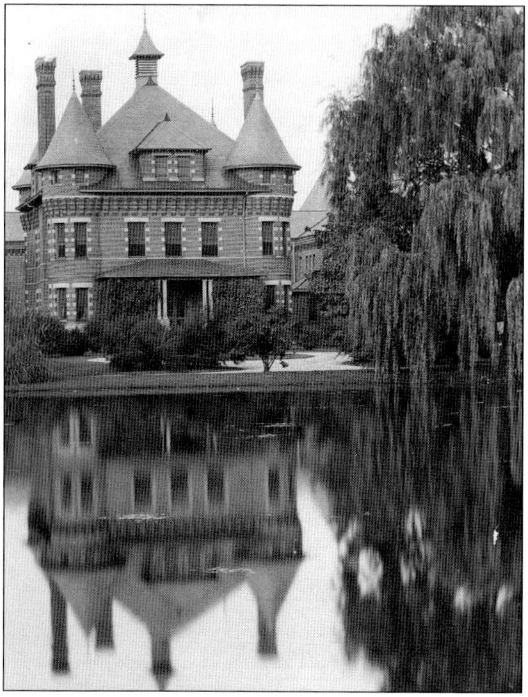

The Women's Strong Ward is reflected in the large lake known as the Sunken Garden. The two strong wards were used for only the severest of cases—the violent, "incurable," and suicidal, for example. Those patients placed in the strong wards were only kept there until they were well enough to be moved to one of the cottages. (TLCPL.)

The Men's Strong Ward was similar in design to the women's building and was located on the opposite end of the hospital grounds. Both structures were physically incorporated into the larger Men's and Women's Hospitals constructed in the late 19th and early 20th centuries. Originally, the two strong wards were the only buildings on the hospital grounds that had bars on their windows. (TLCPL.)

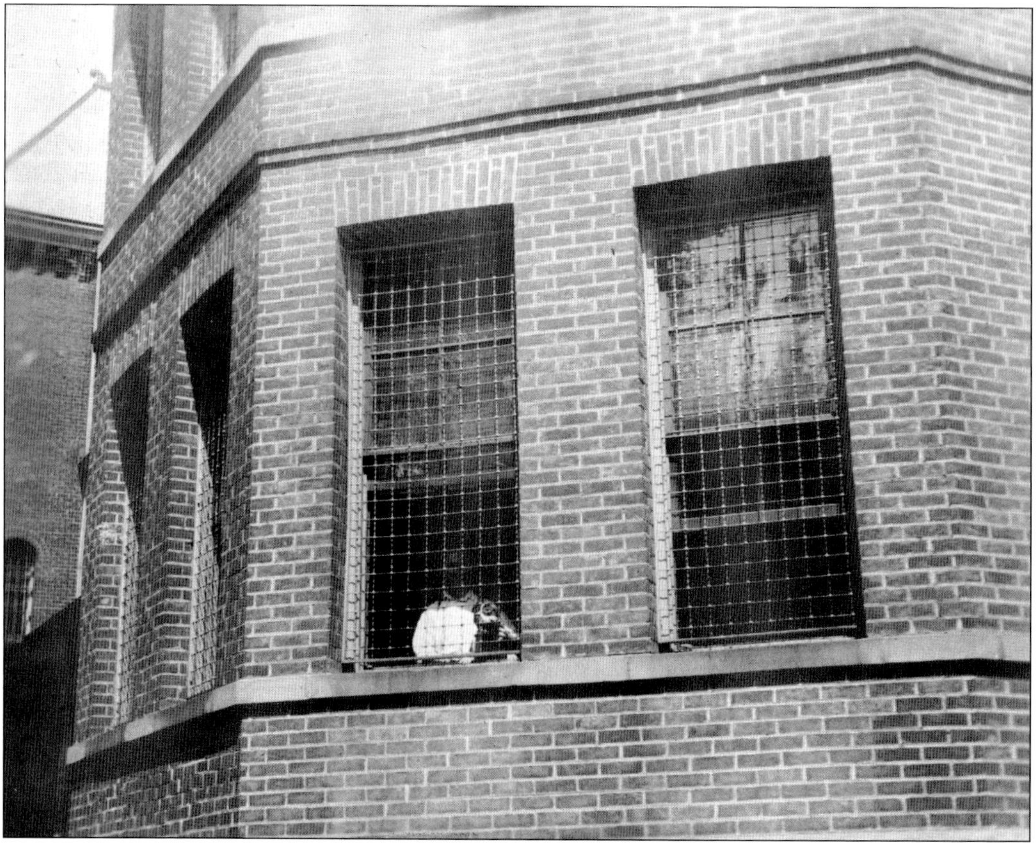

Dr. Frederick Arthur Todd was only 33 years old when a stray dog wandered onto the hospital grounds. The dog had rabies, and the doctor was bitten. Two patients chased the dog down and killed it, but the doctor later died in a hospital in Chicago. The dog pictured here appears in several photographs with attendants in various spots on the grounds. (TLCPL.)

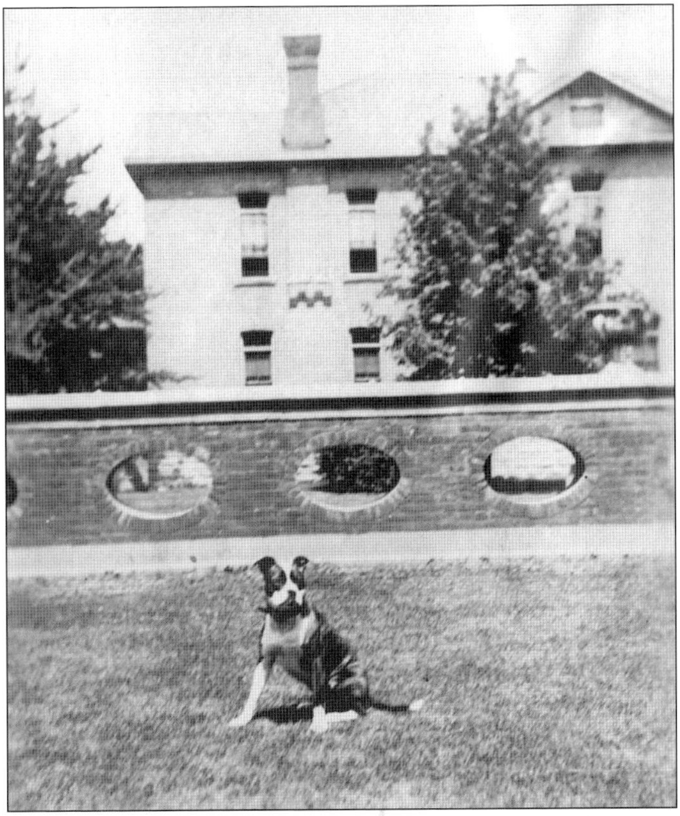

Dogs and cats appear in many of the hospital photographs with attendants and patients, and near patient areas. Here, a man and woman show off the tricks their dog can do, with patients watching from the Women's Hospital Annex behind them. Having pets around the hospitals and cottages likely had some therapeutic value. (NOPH.)

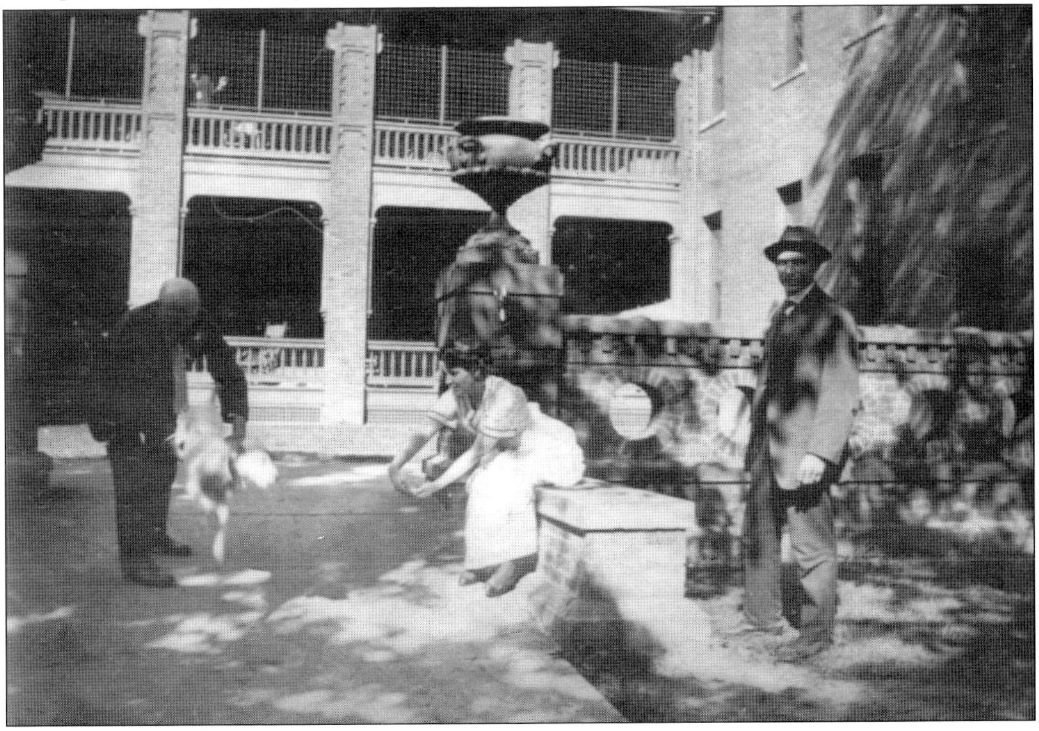

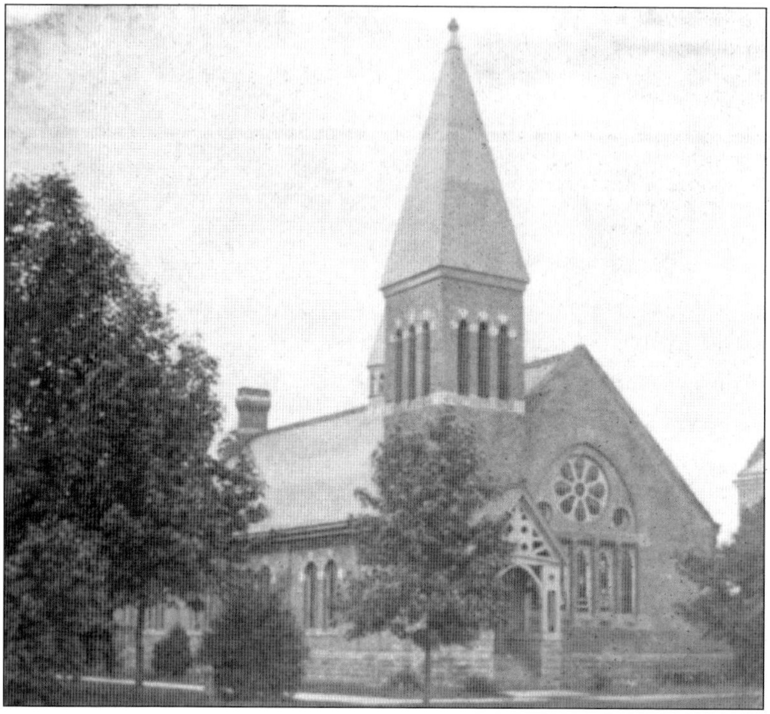

The chapel was one of the original 34 buildings constructed in 1888. It was used for interdenominational worship, funerals, and even a few weddings. Religious services were held twice a week, and patients were encouraged to attend as part of their therapy. By 1920, its Protestant congregation outgrew the building, and it was used for occupational therapy classes. (NOPH.)

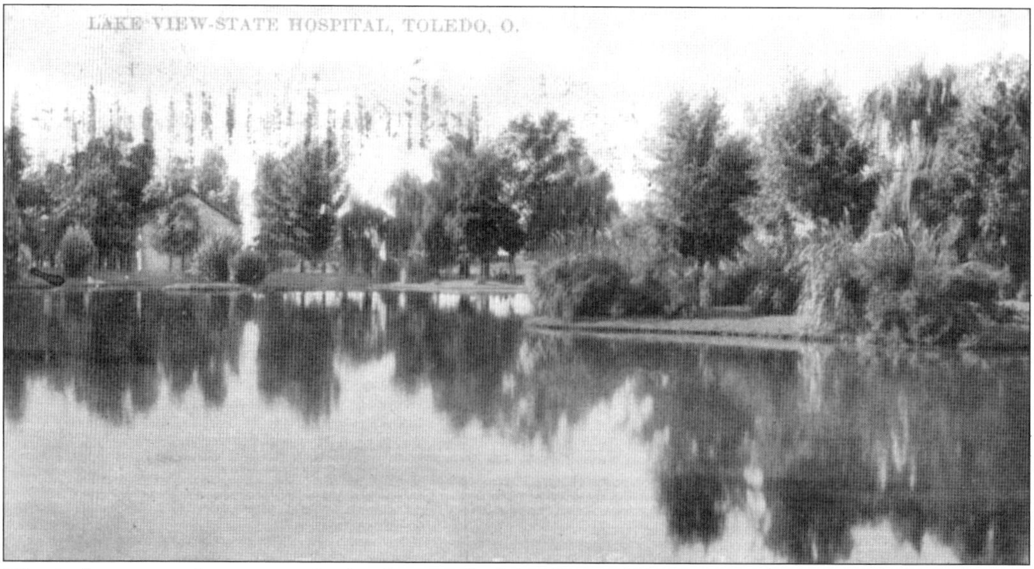

The icehouse can be seen in the background of this beautiful scene on the hospital's largest lake. Ice was harvested from this lake in the winter and stored in this building for use in the summer, thus its close proximity to the lake. The walls of the icehouse were insulated with sawdust. (NOPH.)

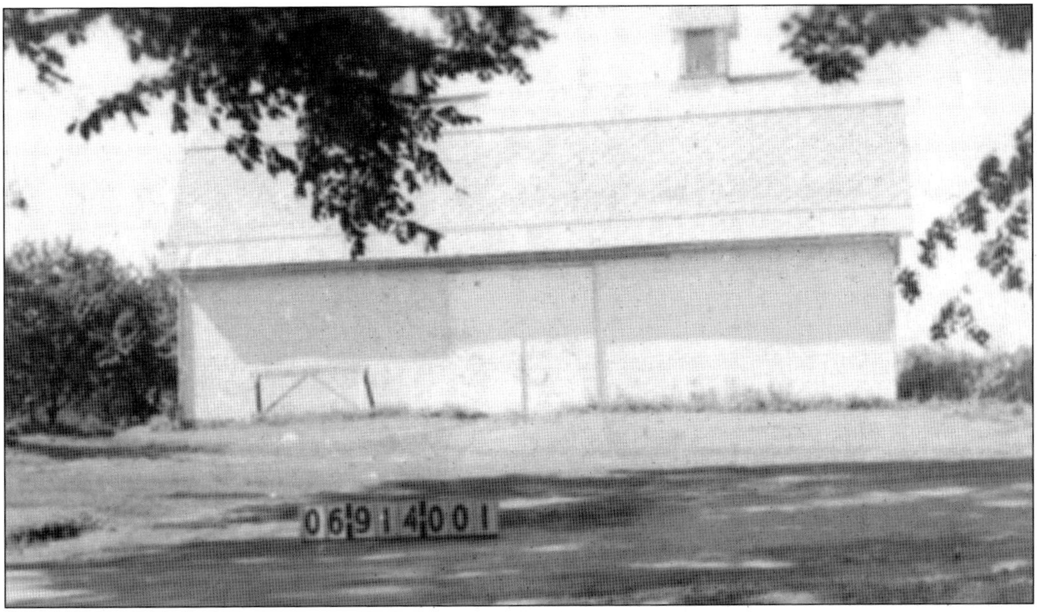

The farm operation supplemented the hospital's food supply and provided a great source of occupational therapy. By 1899, male patients, many of whom were experienced farmers and gardeners, were cultivating 240 acres of fruits, vegetables, and other crops. This was one of the earliest barns on the property and was located on the north side of Arlington Avenue. (TLCPL.)

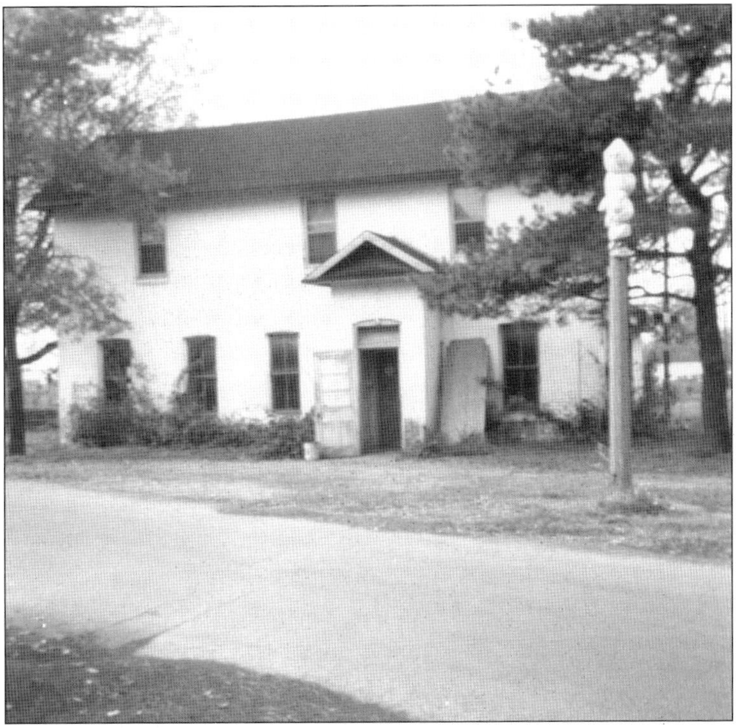

The greenhouse was built in 1893. Here, skilled patients propagated plants for later transfer to the hospital's landscape, gardens, and fields. Flowers and potted plants were also produced for decorating the wards and filling the giant urns that graced the hospital's grounds. The building was soon expanded to meet the need for more plants as the hospital grew and the cultivated acreage increased. (NOPH.)

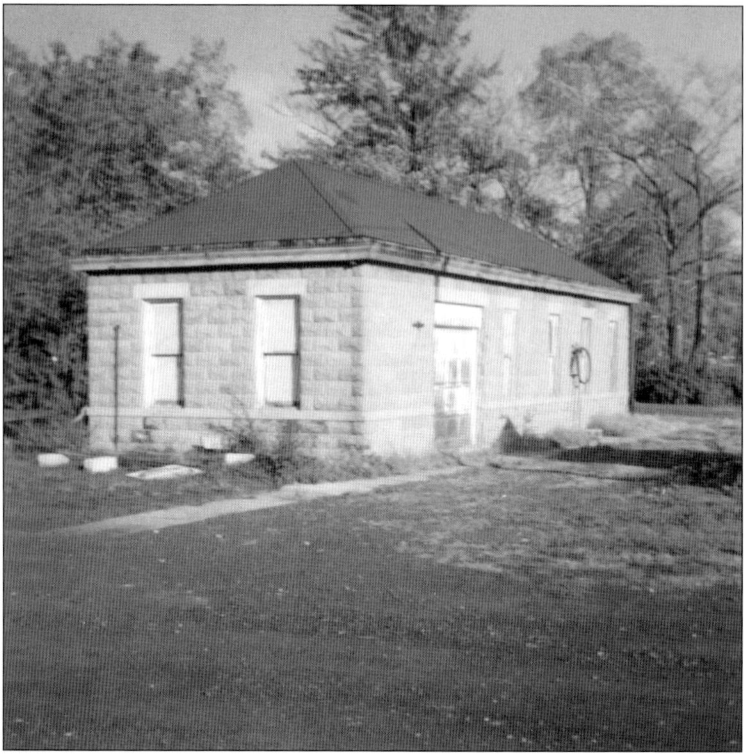

Around 1905, hog pens and fences were added to the farm, making it possible for patients to produce pork to supplement the hospital's meat supply. Pictured here is the blacksmith shop. Other early farm buildings included the farm office, kraut house, storage building, and the barn known as the White Barn. Many more buildings were constructed later as the farm expanded its operations. (NOPH.)

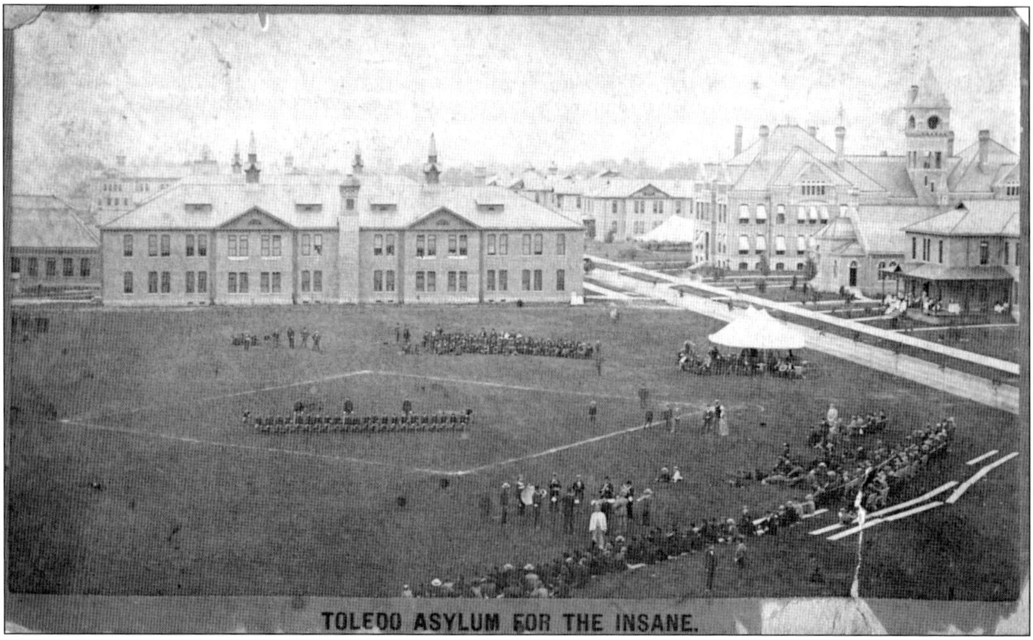

Baseball and other competitive sports were a source of diversion for the troubled mind. Here, teams, spectators, and dignitaries gather for a game on the recreation field, as patients and attendants sit on porches ready to watch around 1890. A brass band provides pre-game entertainment, and tents for other activities add to the festive atmosphere. In the background is one of the dining halls. (TLCPL.)

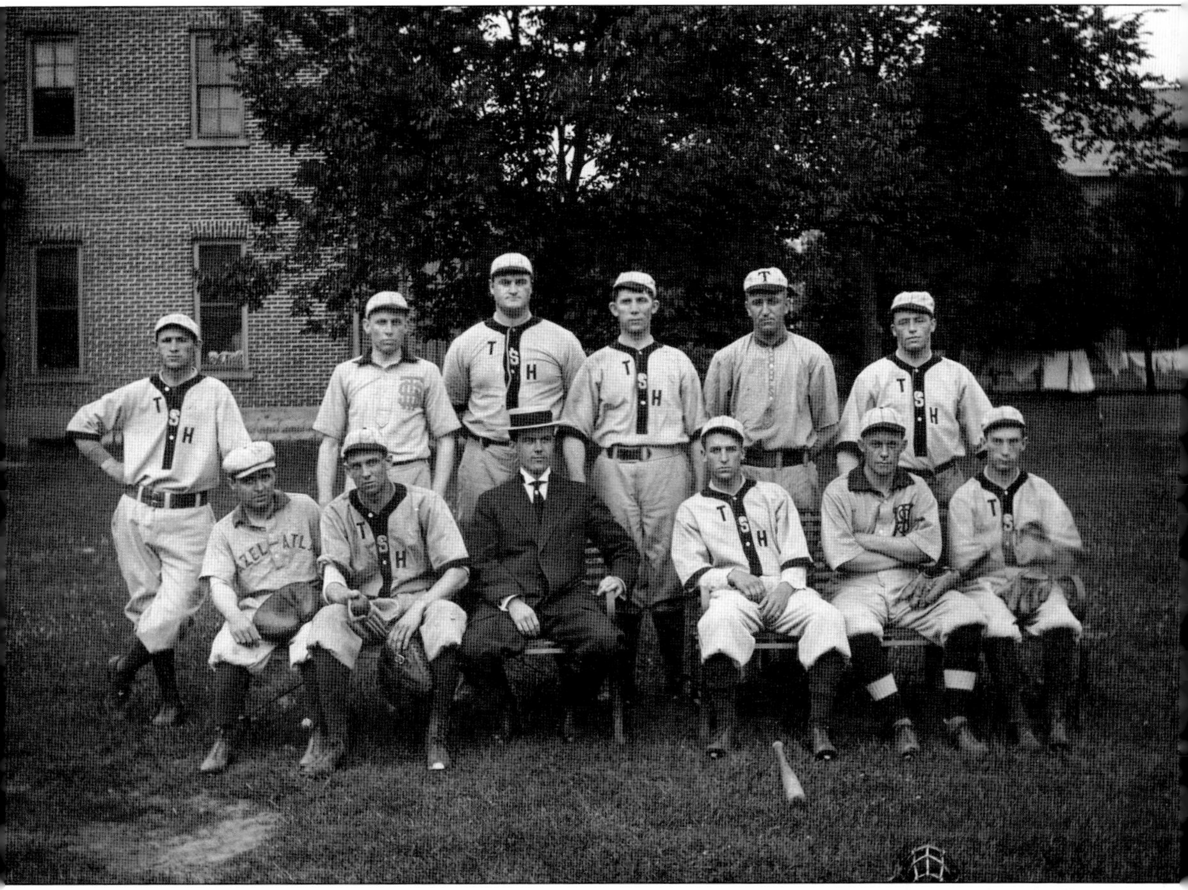

The hospital's baseball team, made up of both patients and staff, was said to be the best baseball team in northwest Ohio. Games between the hospital team and other teams around the area were one form of therapeutic recreation provided to the hospital's patients and staff. Note their mismatched uniforms. (TLCPL.)

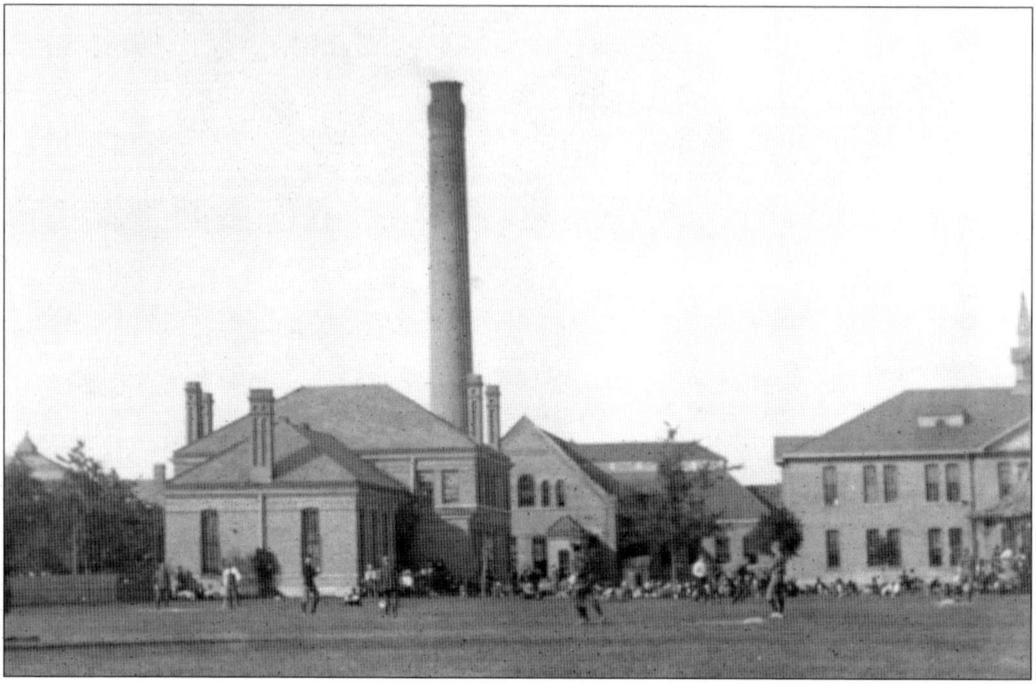

In 1897, the hospital's team won 31 out of 36 games played on the hospital grounds. One of the games lost that year, against the YMCA's Outing Club, was reported to be "a close and exciting game . . . one of the best games played on the asylum grounds this season." (NOPH.)

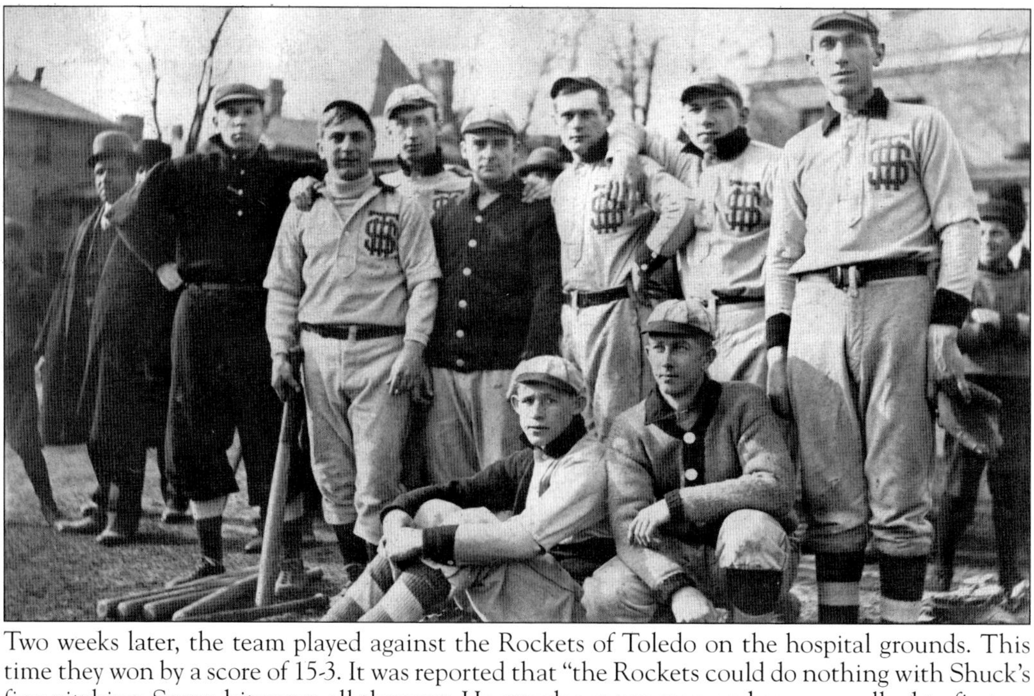

Two weeks later, the team played against the Rockets of Toledo on the hospital grounds. This time they won by a score of 15-3. It was reported that "the Rockets could do nothing with Shuck's fine pitching. Seven hits were all they got. He struck out ten men and no one walked to first on balls." The pitcher was William C. Shuck, a hospital attendant. (TLCPL.)

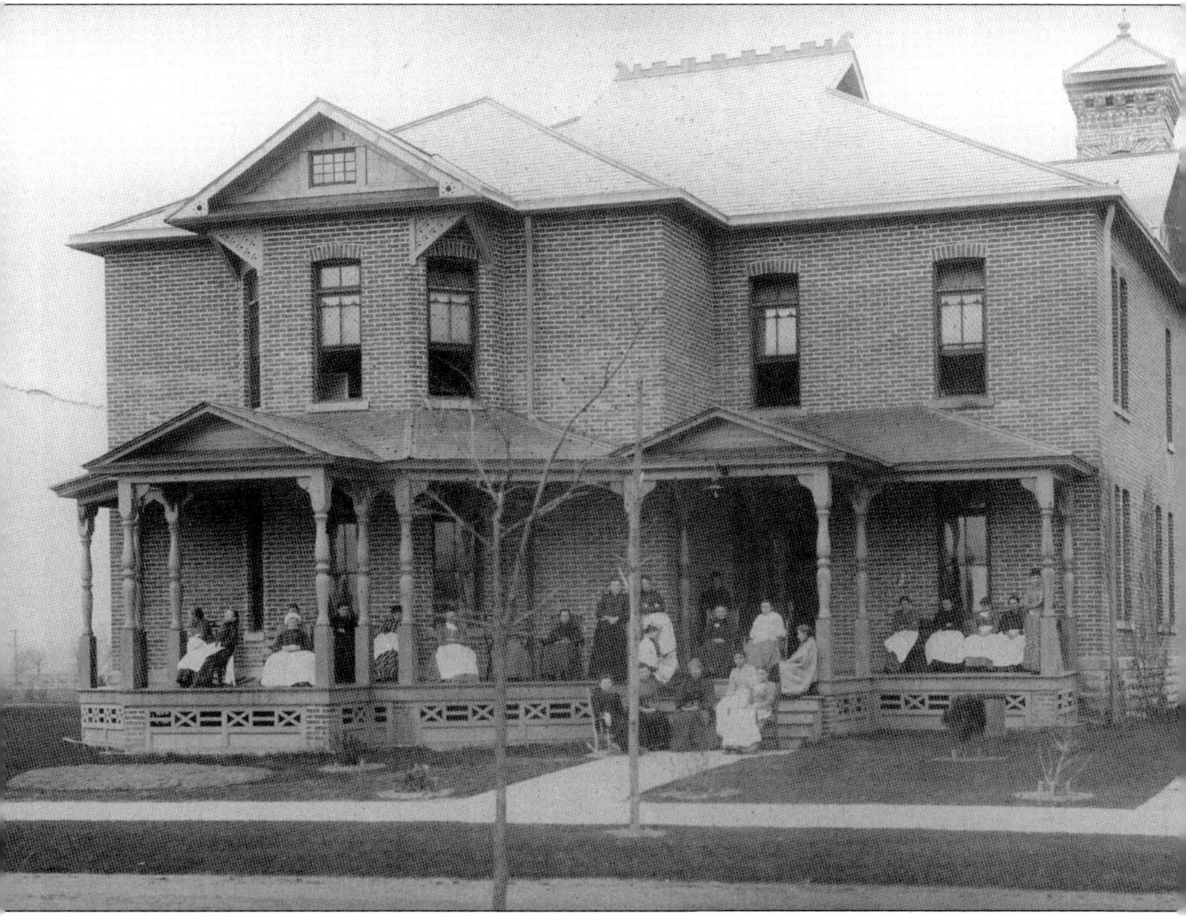

Some causes of insanity recorded in patient records in the early years were "religious excitement," "intemperance in drink," "domestic trouble," "financial trouble," "sexual self-abuse," "love affairs," "puberty," "cigarettes," and "changes of life." Forms of mental disease listed included "insanity of pregnancy," "pubescent and adolescent," "drug habit," and "puerperal mania." (TLCPL.)

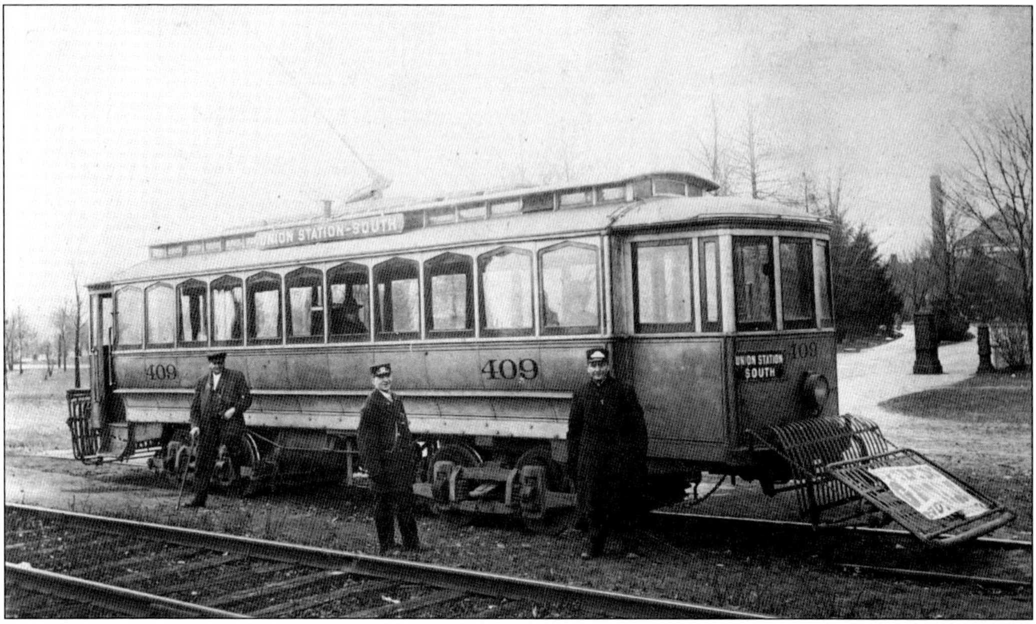

Streetcars were a popular form of transportation for Toledoans in the late 19th and early 20th centuries. Car No. 419 of the Toledo Railway & Light Company line provided service from downtown Toledo to the state hospital. This photograph shows the car at the main entrance to the hospital, the end of the line. (TLCPL.)

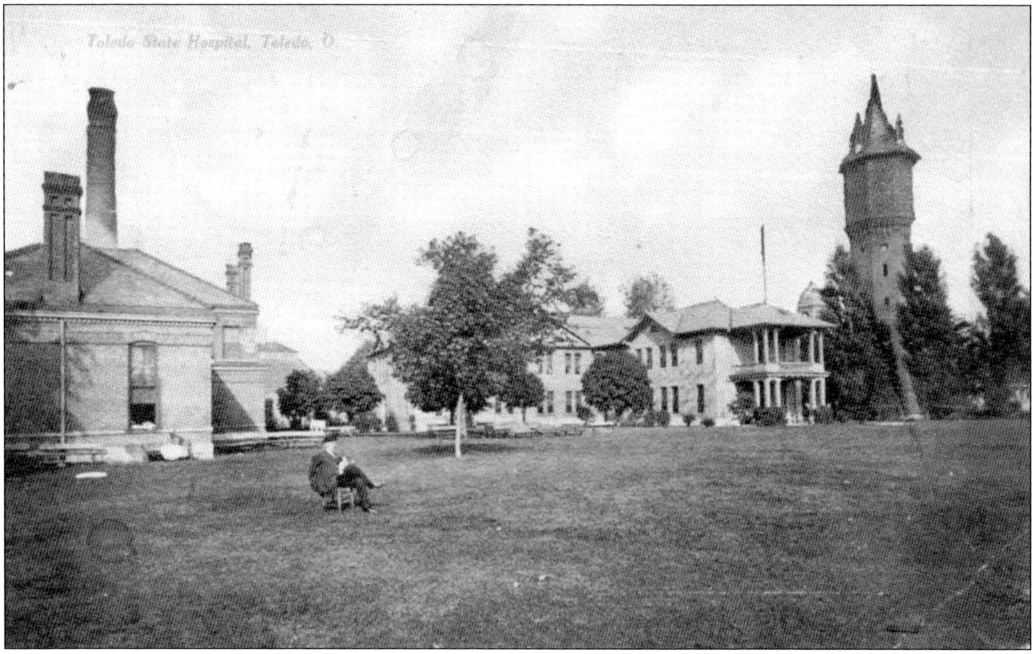

Among the occupations of male patients admitted to the hospital in 1904 were blacksmith, bricklayer, physician, teacher, musician, soldier, and lawyer. Whether by disease, traumatic brain injury, age-related illness, environmental influences, or genetics, this abbreviated list demonstrates that anyone can become "insane" at any given time and that mental illness does not discriminate as to race, class, religion, profession, or origin. (TLCPL.)

Vaudeville and burlesque performer Jennie Dickerson became a patient in 1892 after others in her troupe noticed her "mental unbalance" during performances at a Cincinnati vaudeville house. While confined at the hospital, she began writing poetry, and her work was published in four volumes. At that time, private social welfare groups were forming all around the country, and a group of Cleveland businessmen had formed a society to help unfortunates who showed talent in one of the arts. They took an interest in Jennie's poetry, particularly one poem entitled, "The Dream Worlds." In 1910, they wrote to hospital administrators asking that Jennie be released to their care. They intended to find a suitable private home for her, contingent on her doctors' approval. She was not discharged, however, until 1916. What became of her after that is unknown. (Both, NOPH.)

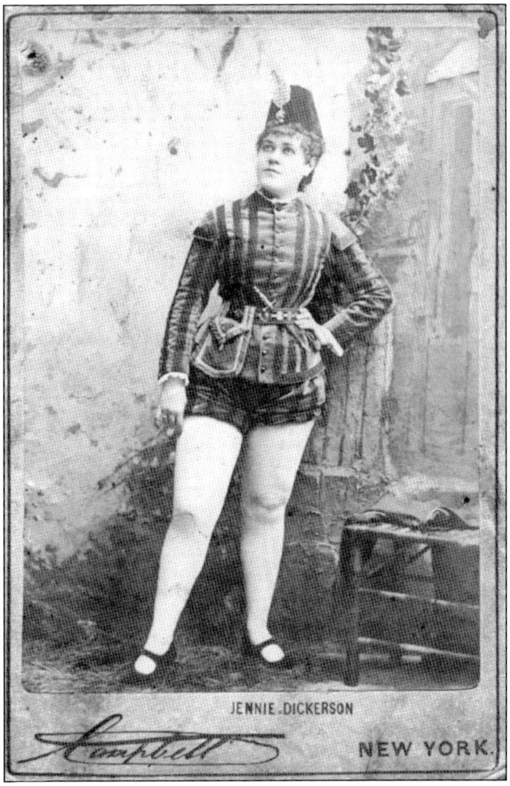

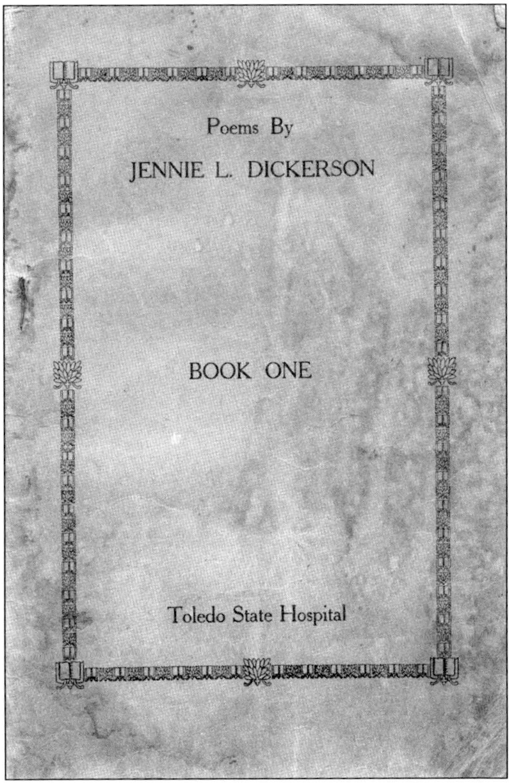
Poems By

JENNIE L. DICKERSON

BOOK ONE

Toledo State Hospital

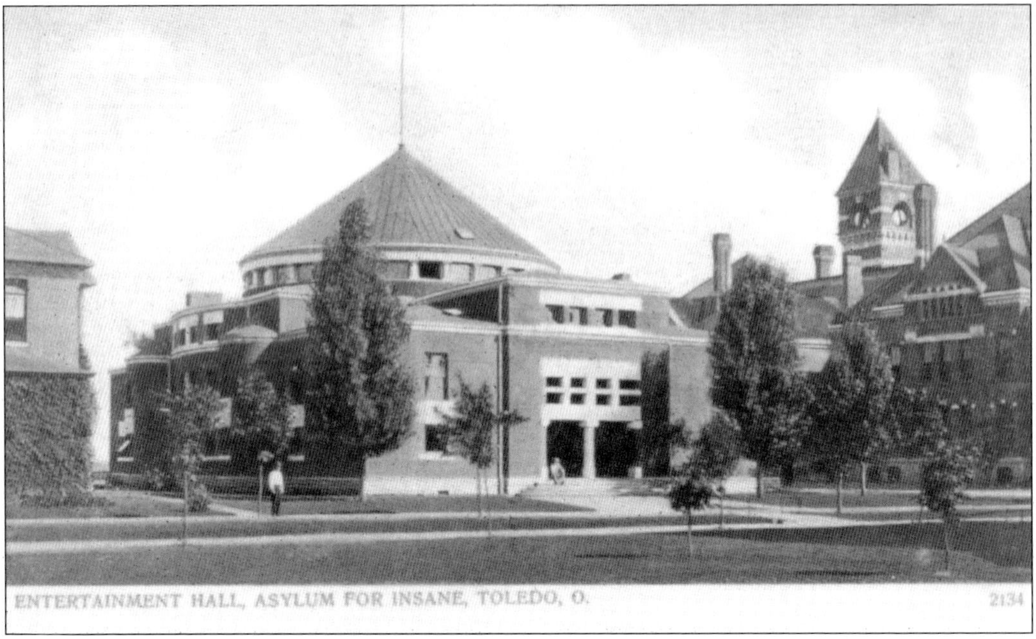

The Entertainment Hall was added in 1890. It held weekly dances, masquerade balls, concerts, theatrical performances, "sleight of hand" shows, movies, and other amusements. Dr. Tobey wrote, "Every effort has been put forth to occupy both the time and attention of the inmates in a natural and wholesome way." The hall was later used for Protestant church services. Catholic services were held in the chapel. (NOPH.)

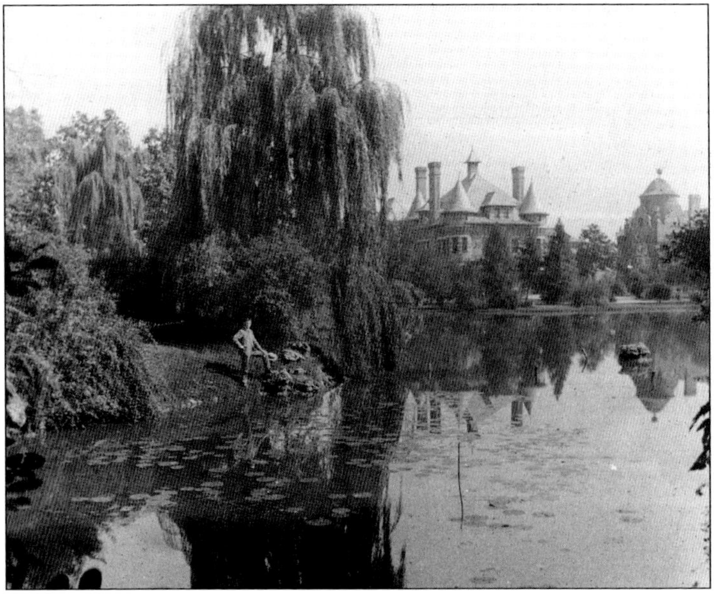

A brief, politically motivated interruption in Dr. Tobey's tenure as superintendent occurred in 1891, when Dr. C.E. Tupper, "a country doctor, well advanced in years and without experience in the treatment of the insane," was appointed to replace him. The appointment was influenced by Tupper's son-in-law, who was on Gov. James E. Campbell's (1890–1892) staff. Dr. Tobey was reappointed immediately after the new governor, William McKinley, took office in 1892. (TLCPL.)

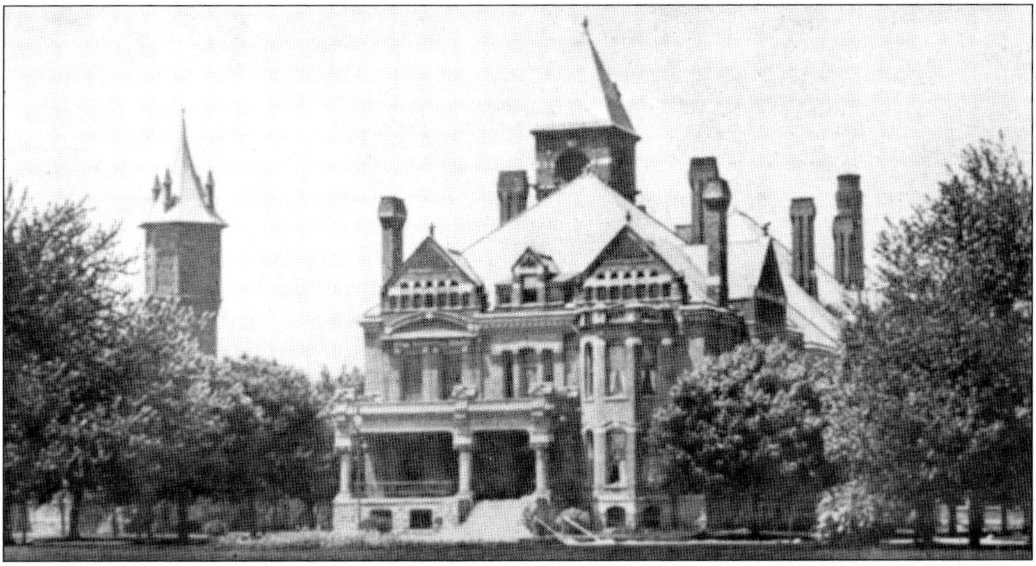

In 1894, the hospital's name was changed from the Toledo Asylum for the Insane to the Toledo State Hospital. While the word "asylum" means a place of safety or sanctuary, by the 19th century it had developed a negative meaning because of poor conditions and frightening treatment methods often found in hospitals for the mentally ill. (NOPH.)

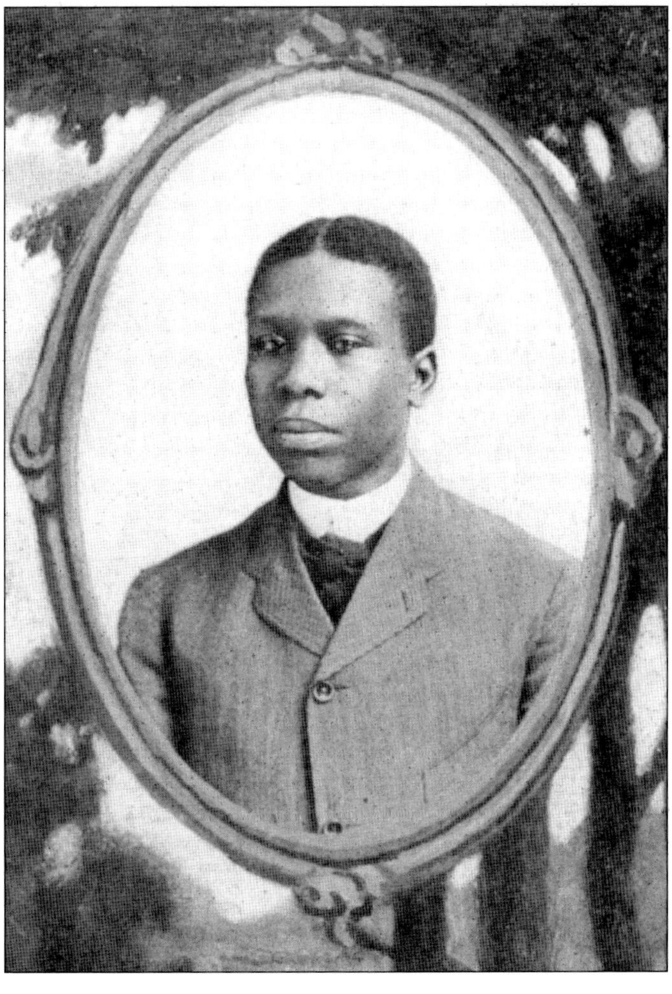

In 1895, Dr. Tobey was introduced to poet Paul Laurence Dunbar, and the two became fast friends. Dunbar often visited Tobey at the state hospital and returned several times to read his poems for patients, employees, and local dignitaries. His poems "Lead Gently" and "The Crisis" were written while visiting the hospital. (NOPH.)

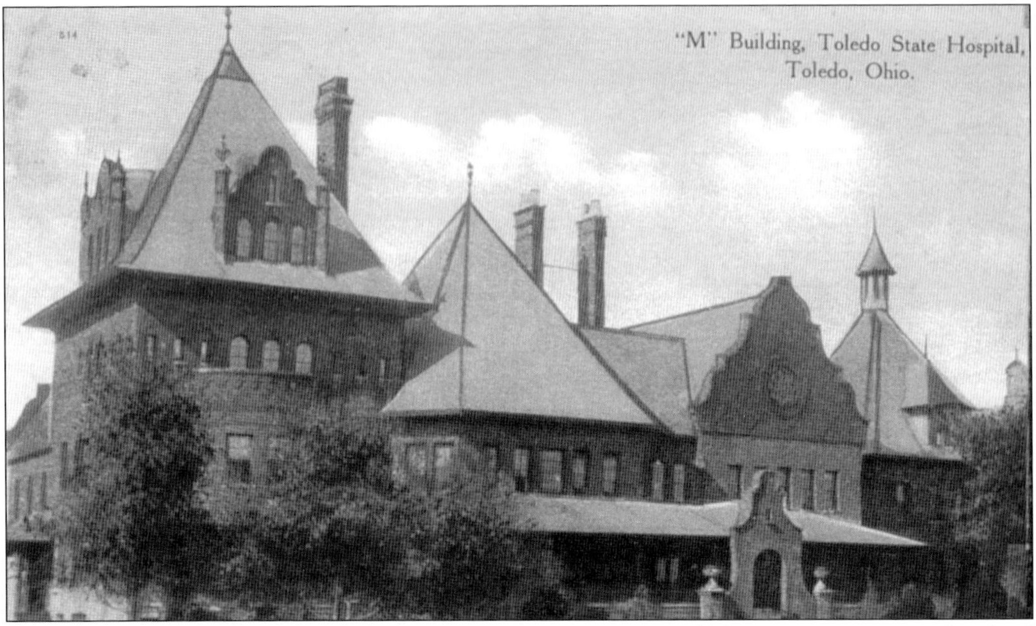

An additional hospital for men was completed in 1899 and could house 80 patients. The third floor of this building was used as a dormitory for male attendants. Around the same time, additions were made to the Men's Strong Ward and several of the men's cottages, increasing the hospital's capacity to 1,600. (NOPH.)

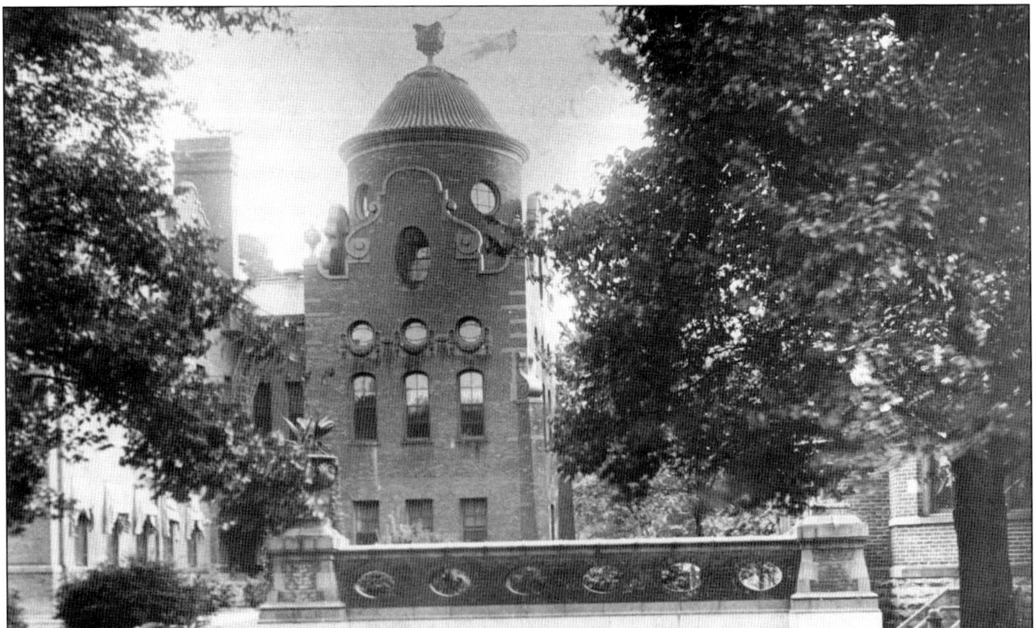

Another hospital for women was constructed in 1901. While the new women's building could accommodate 60 patients, it was still necessary to use the chapel as an additional female ward. In this photograph, the new women's building appears much different than the men's, but they were, in fact, of similar architectural design. (TLCPL.)

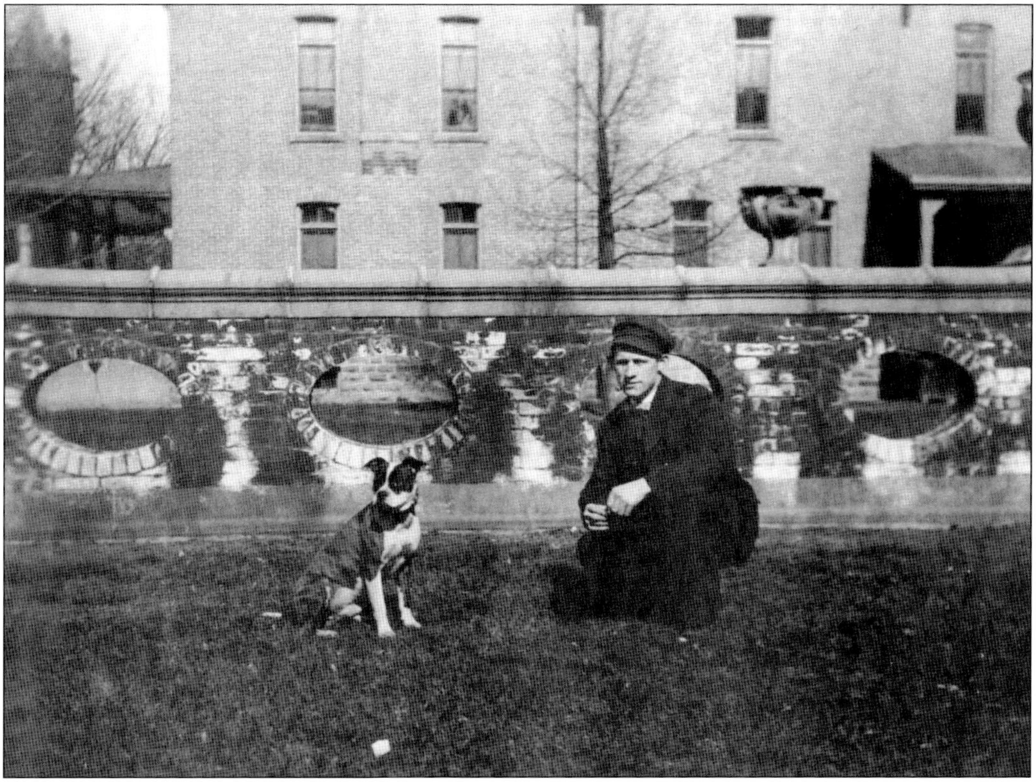

Employees often lived on the grounds alongside their patients, as work shifts were long and travel was difficult. Staff living quarters were set up in some of the cottages and upper floors of other buildings on the hospital grounds. For many, this was an indication of their dedication and commitment to the patients in their care. (TLCPL.)

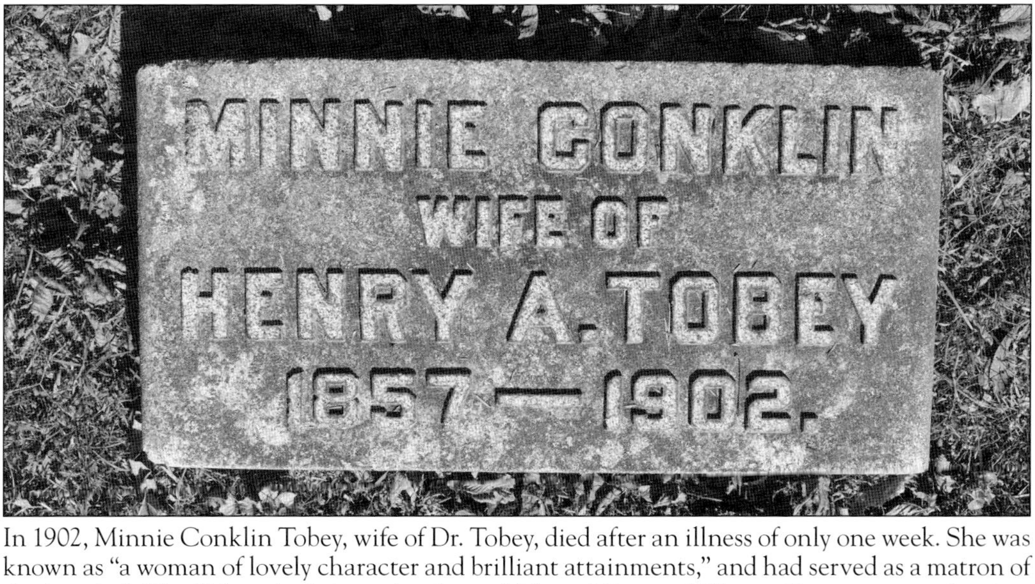

In 1902, Minnie Conklin Tobey, wife of Dr. Tobey, died after an illness of only one week. She was known as "a woman of lovely character and brilliant attainments," and had served as a matron of the hospital. The Tobeys had three daughters, Helen, Alice, and Clara, all teenagers at the time of her death. She is buried at Woodlawn Cemetery in Toledo. (Photograph by author.)

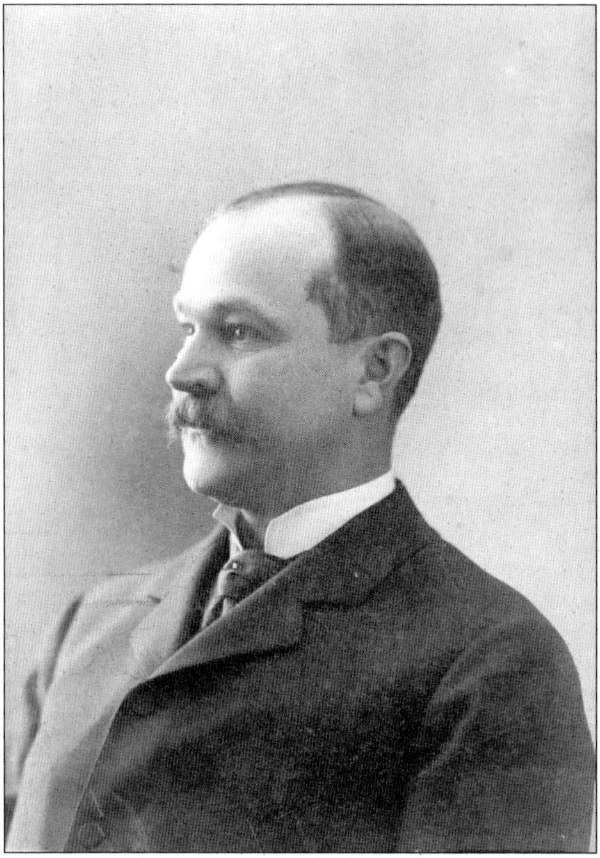

After his wife's death, Dr. Tobey was completely brokenhearted. He began drinking heavily and was eventually unable to carry out his duties effectively. He retired in 1906 and became so ill that he himself was admitted to the state hospital. In 1908, he died suddenly of heart failure while on a fishing trip and was buried alongside his wife. Upon his retirement, the hospital's board of trustees wrote, "The beneficent influence of the faithful, competent and persistent endeavor of this eminent scholar and gentleman, in developing and promoting . . . what is known as the Cottage System, will be felt as a blessing to mankind, and will prove a monument to . . . this kind hearted friend of his race whom the world owes a debt of gratitude and affection." (Left, NOPH; below, photograph by author.)

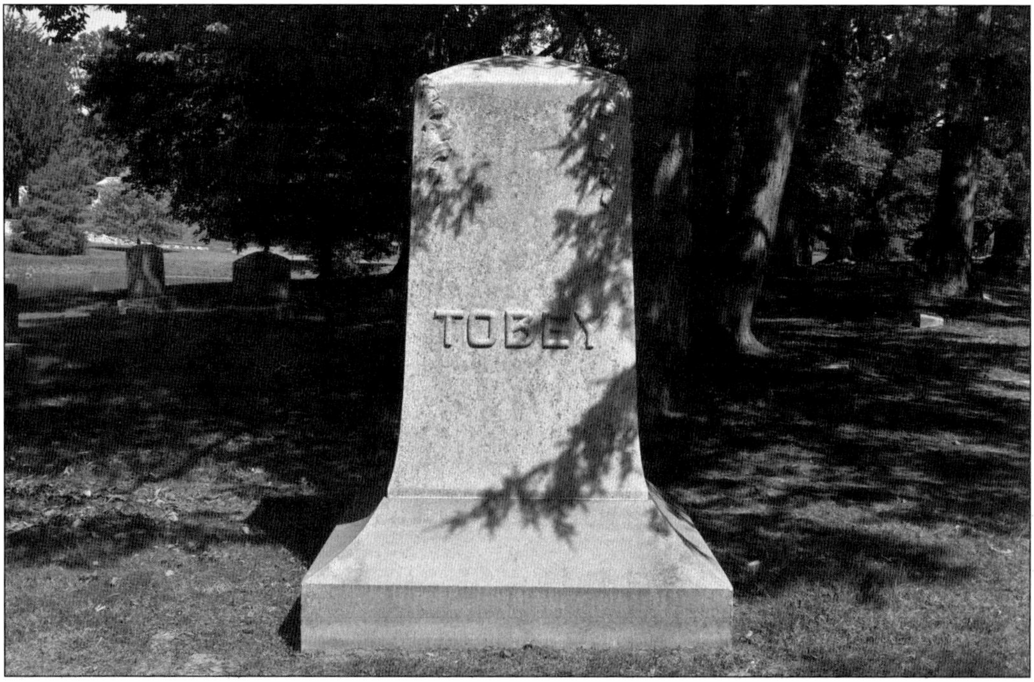

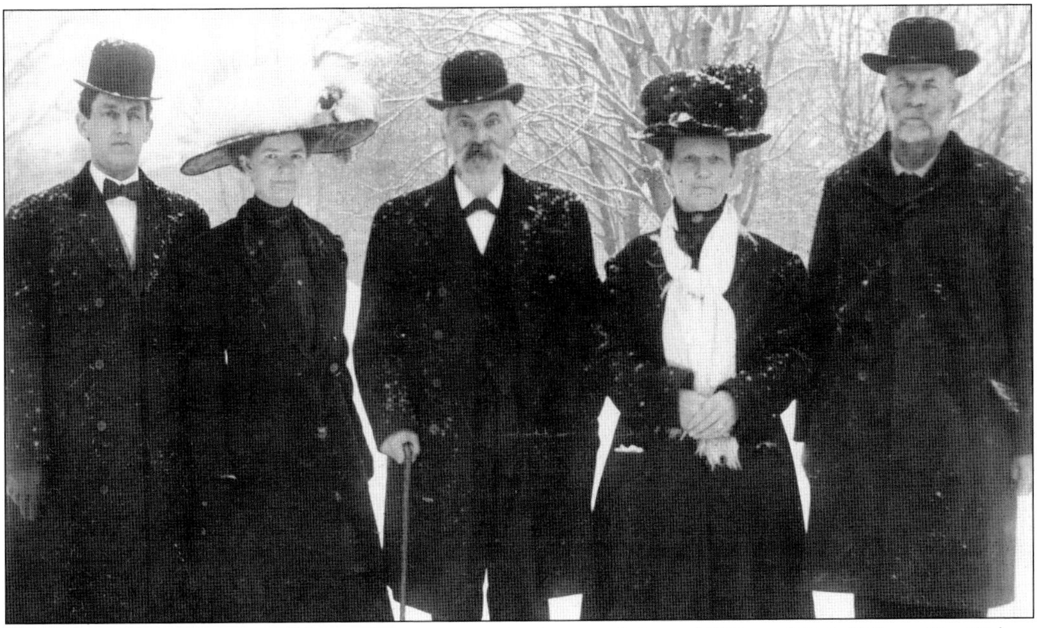

Dr. George R. Love served as a physician at the hospital from 1898 to 1904. When Dr. Tobey retired, Love returned as superintendent and served until 1919. A eugenicist, he supported efforts to improve the human race by preventing the reproduction of individuals with defective or undesirable genetic traits. Whether Dr. Love authorized the sterilization of patients at the hospital is unknown. Pictured here are members of the medical staff around 1920. (NOPH.)

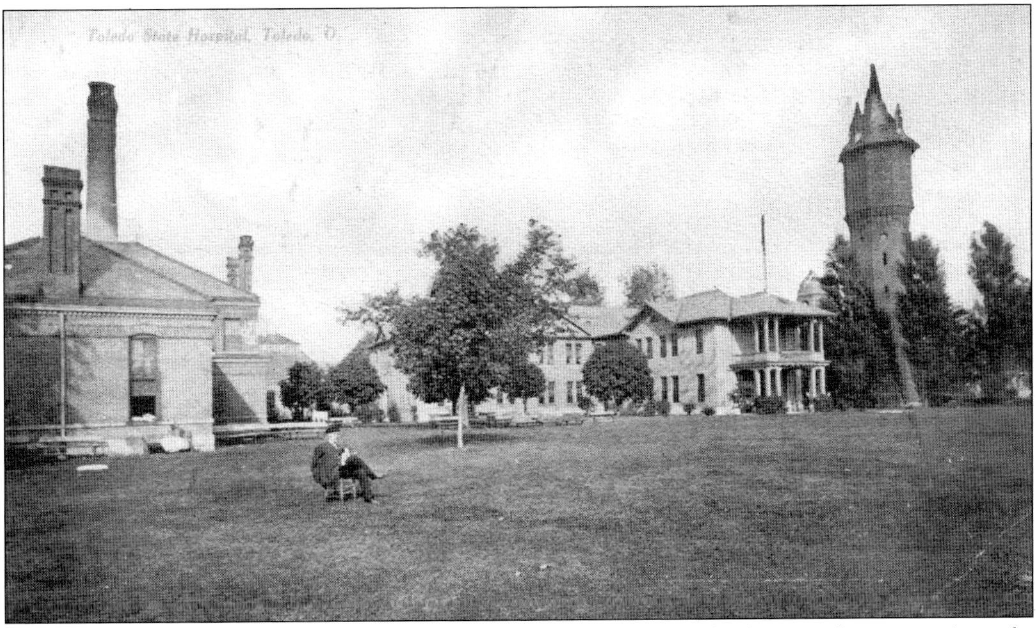

The Occupational Therapy Building, seen here around 1900, had space for women's crafts including dressmaking, general sewing, leatherworking, rug-making, painting, and papercrafts, and a room for storing clothing made by patients. Women also did needlework and created other artistic works. In later years, Ida Fordyce, wife of Supt. O.O. Fordyce, taught art classes here for female patients. (NOPH.)

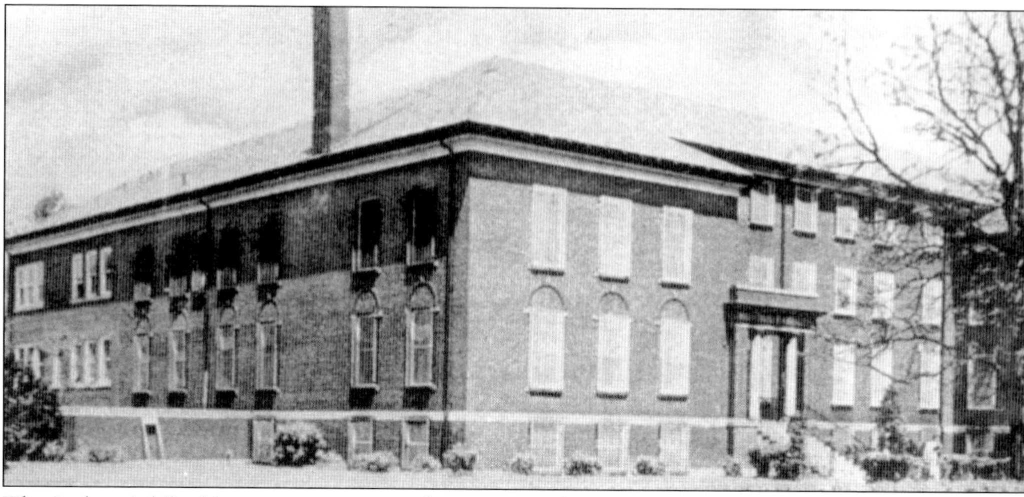

The Industrial Building was constructed in 1908 and was used for men's occupational therapy. It was here that male patients built and refinished furniture, did upholstery, wicker, and woodwork and engaged in other skilled crafts. The hospital gift shop was also located in this building at one time, and it was later used for an employee residence. (NOPH.)

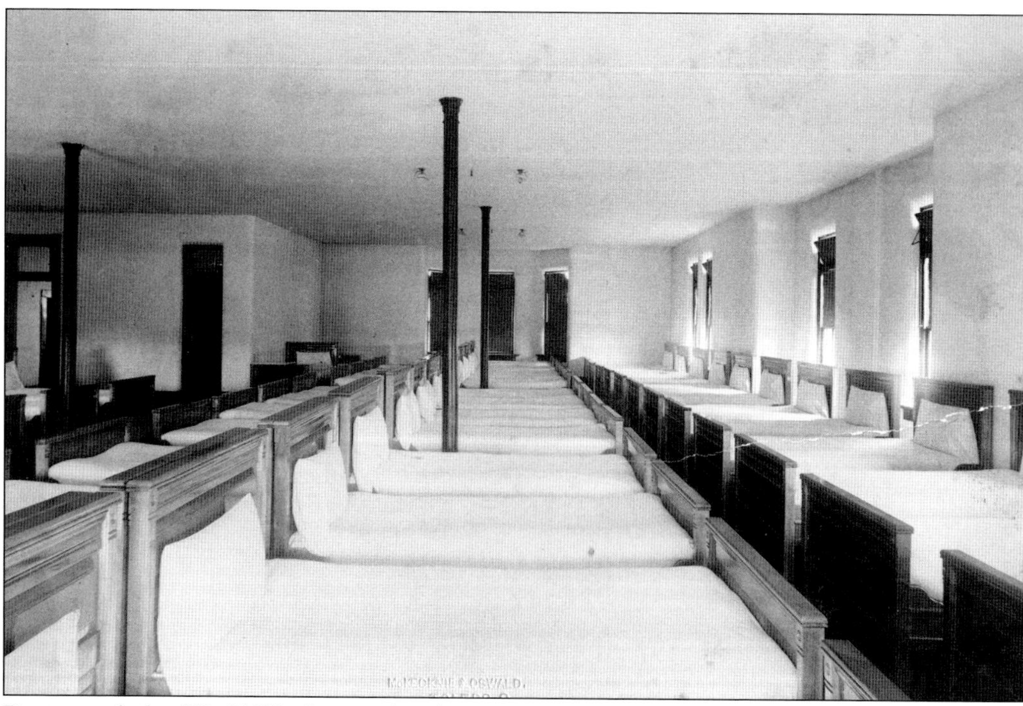

During and after World War I, war-related issues caused an increase in admissions. Also, a change in admission policies allowed individuals to commit themselves and circumvent the court system. This encouraged individuals and families to seek help for their loved ones for the first time. These events, along with improvements in treatment methods, led to the first of many overcrowding issues to come. (TLCPL.)

In the years following 1917, a better informed and educated public resulted in an increase in awareness of mental illness. Families and friends were faced with how to help loved ones returning from war cope with difficult physical injuries and emotional issues. Treatment options available to doctors at that time were hydrotherapy, occupational therapy, recreational therapy, malarial therapy, and medication. (TLCPL.)

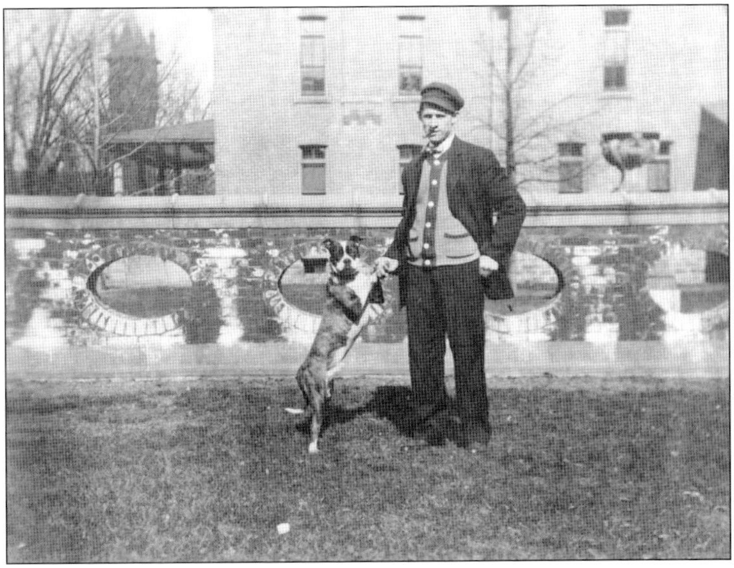

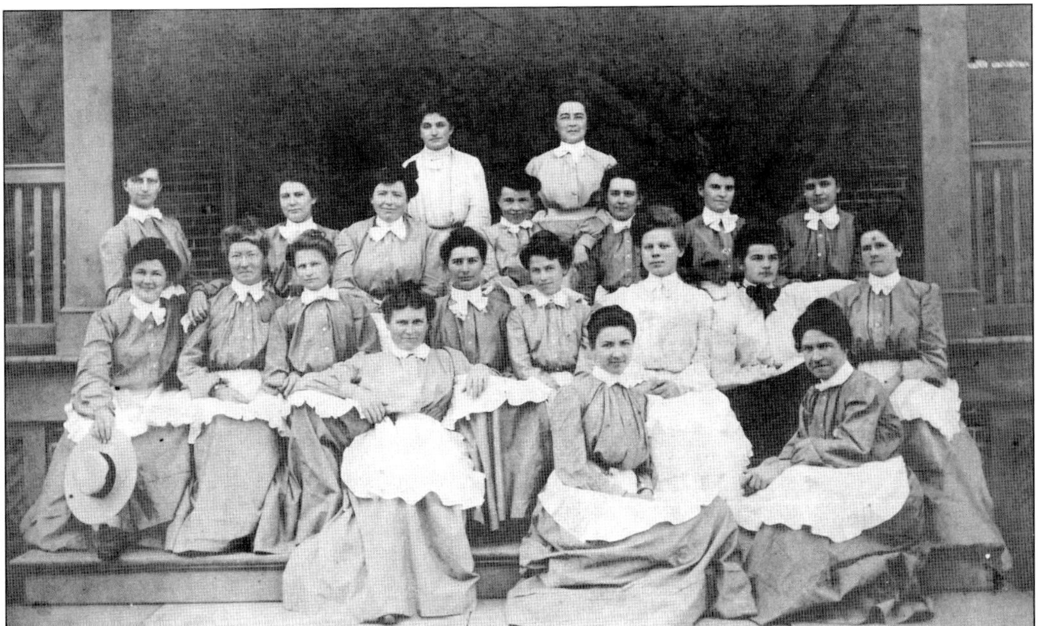

In 1919, a two-year nurse's training school was organized in conjunction with the Lucas County Hospital. Students attended lectures and classes at the county hospital but did clinicals and specialized classwork in psychiatric nursing at the state hospital. The program was eventually expanded to three years and became fully accredited. (TLCPL.)

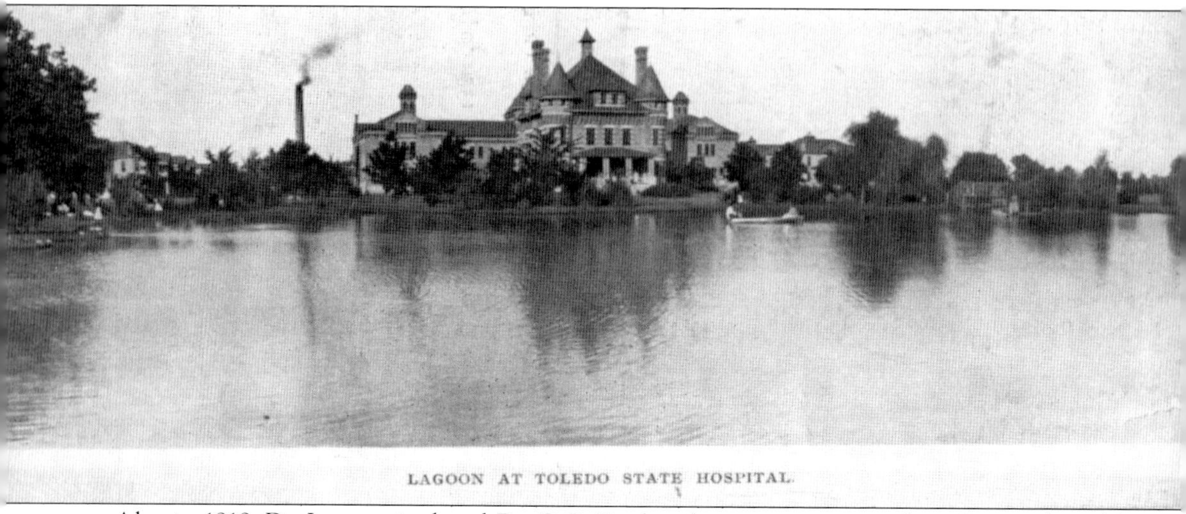

Also in 1919, Dr. Love retired and Dr. O.O. Fordyce became superintendent. Dr. Fordyce, like Dr. Love, was a supporter of eugenics. He wrote that hereditary mental defects and diseases were the least curable and the main cause of overcrowding of the state's institutions and advocated for sterilization laws. Dr. Fordyce had served as superintendent at Athens State Hospital for 10 years prior to moving to Toledo. (NOPH.)

Three

1920–1950

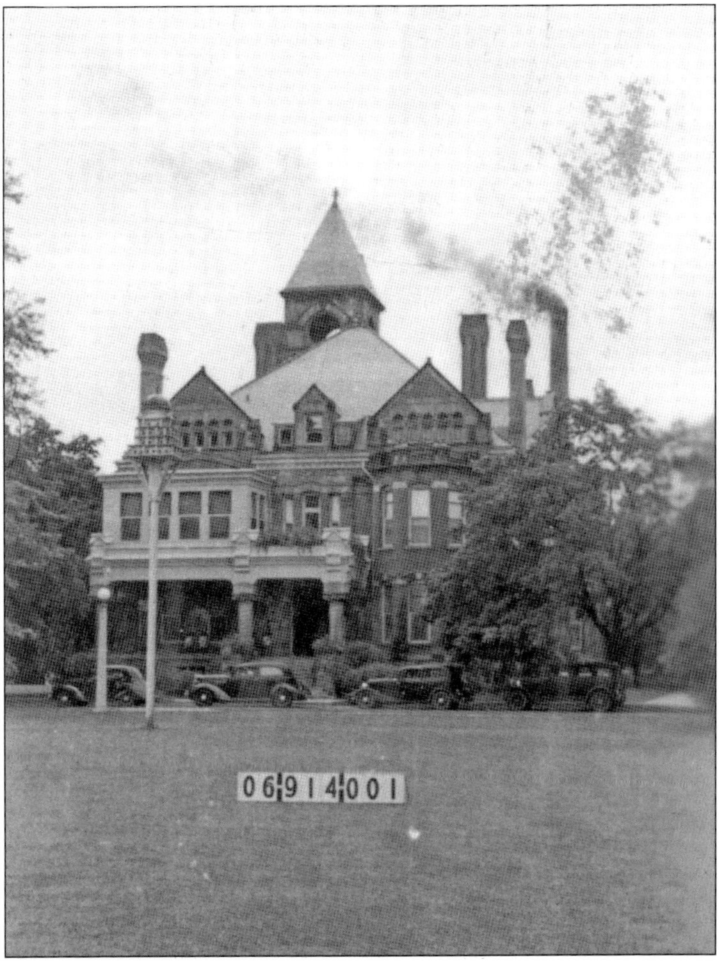

During the next three decades, another world war was fought, the Great Depression wreaked financial devastation, and changes brought on by industrialization were still being felt. The hospital faced staff shortages and chronic overcrowding. However, new medications, improved treatment methods, and the expansion of services helped it meet and even exceed its community's needs. The Administration Building is pictured here around 1930. (TLCPL.)

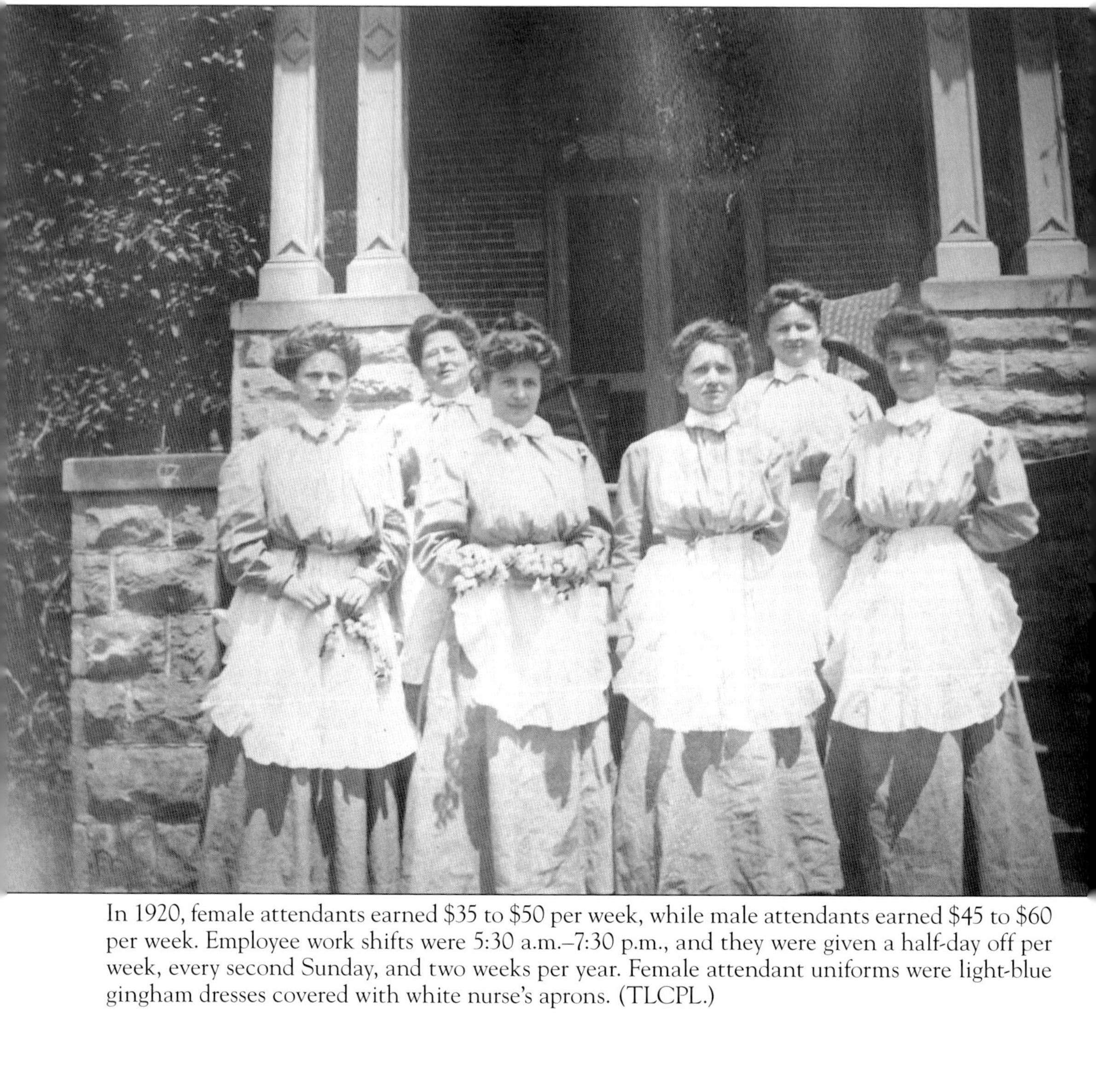

In 1920, female attendants earned $35 to $50 per week, while male attendants earned $45 to $60 per week. Employee work shifts were 5:30 a.m.–7:30 p.m., and they were given a half-day off per week, every second Sunday, and two weeks per year. Female attendant uniforms were light-blue gingham dresses covered with white nurse's aprons. (TLCPL.)

Hydrotherapy equipment first came to the hospital in 1922. Many types were used, including warm baths, hot and cold sprays, and wet sheet wraps. Warm water was used to calm the agitated patient or to relax the insomniac, while cold water was used to invigorate the depressed. Treatments could last for hours or even days. Hydrotherapy was not often used because it was time-consuming and not very effective. (NOPH.)

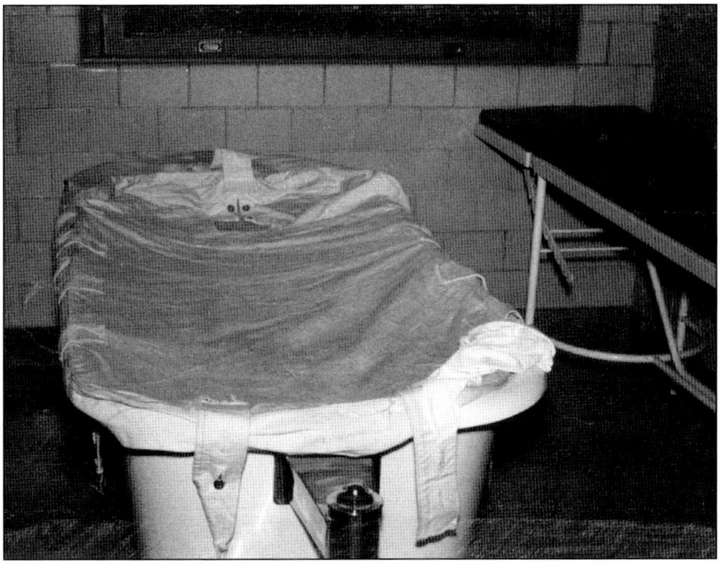

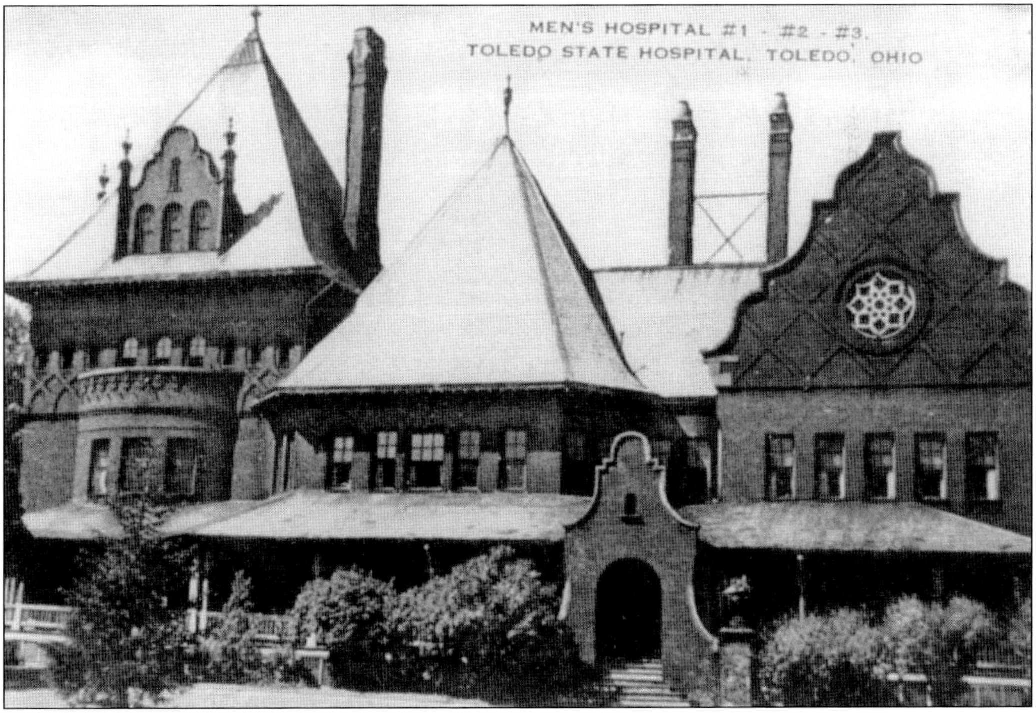

Prior to the discovery of penicillin, syphilis was a major cause of insanity. In 1925, the hospital added a neurosyphilis clinic. Neurosyphilis is the bacterial infection that attacks the brain when syphilis goes untreated. At that time, doctors used a drug called tryparsamide to kill the syphilis bacteria in hopes of preventing the disease from progressing. (NOPH.)

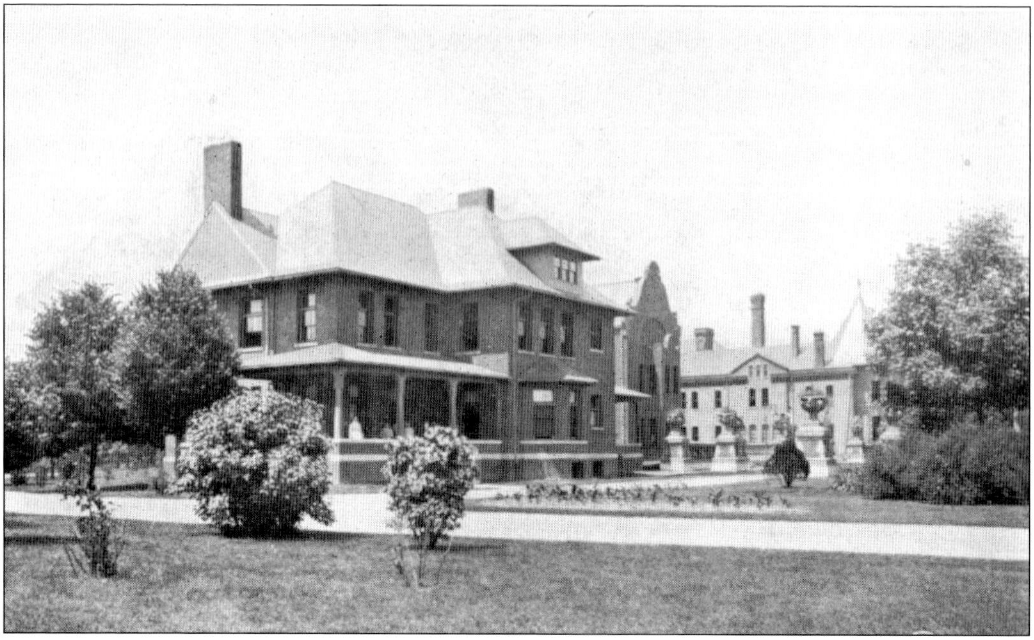

Diagnostic and mental hygiene clinics were also opened around this time. All incoming patients were given a complete physical and mental examination upon admission and diagnosed for treatment. Mental hygiene is the term used to cover all efforts to keep the mind healthy and emphasizes prevention and a proactive approach to illness. (TLCPL.)

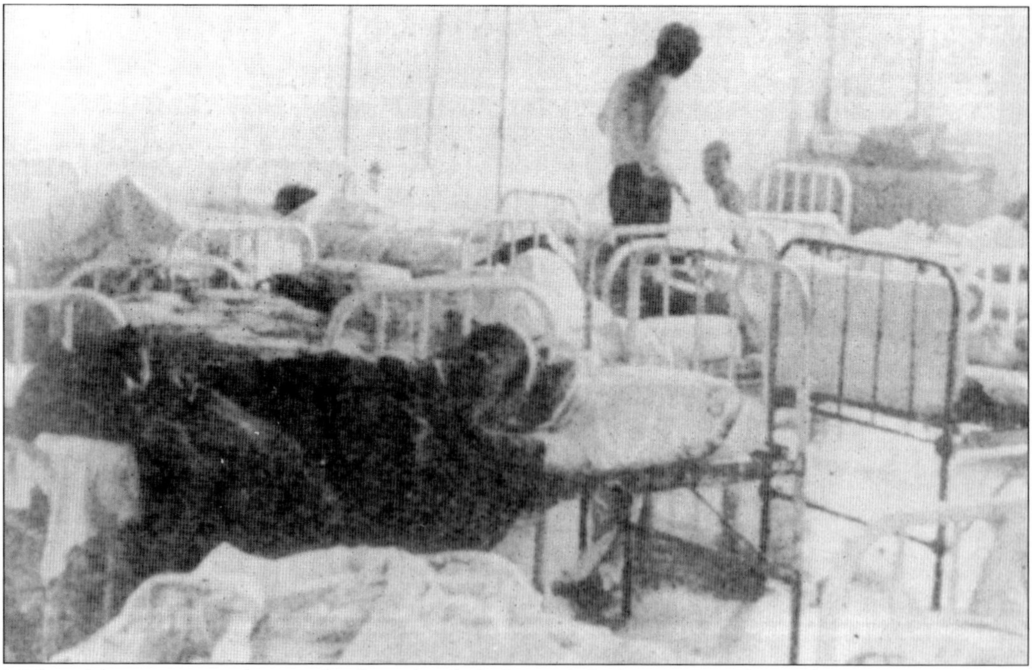

Malarial fever was another method used to kill the syphilis bacteria in the early stages of infection, and in 1925, the hospital opened a malarial therapy clinic. This treatment involved injecting the patient with infected blood in order to induce a high fever (106–108 degrees). If the patient survived the fever, it was likely that they would be cured of syphilis. (NOPH.)

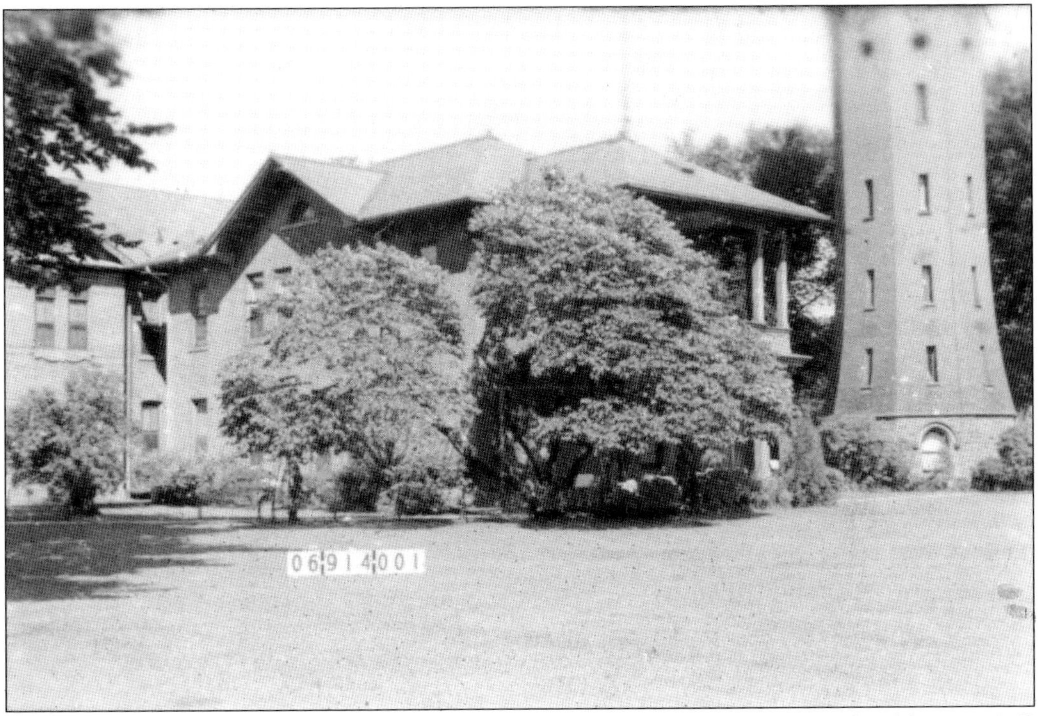

At Dr. Fordyce's urging, a beauty shop was installed in the Occupational Therapy Building in 1925. It was operated by a nurse who had formal training in beauty culture, and two patient assistants. The "Marcel" was the popular hairstyle of the day. In later years, there was also a dedicated space for the women's auxiliary's meetings and projects in this building. (TLCPL.)

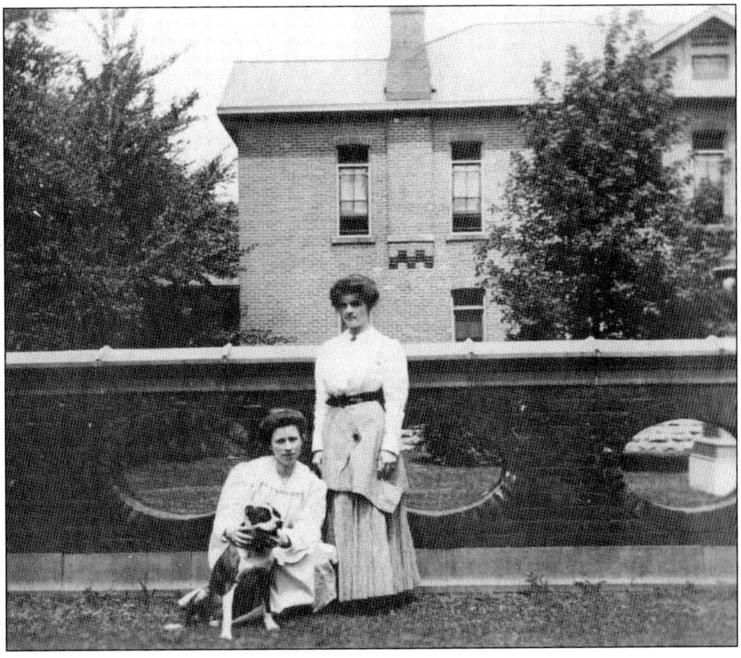

By the 1920s, recreational therapy at the hospital included classes in exercise, calisthenics, hikes, and outdoor sports. Dr. Fordyce believed in recreation as a tool for healing the mind and emphasized, "The circulation is quickened and more blood and nourishment are carried to the brain cells, thereby favoring repair and mental development." (TLCPL.)

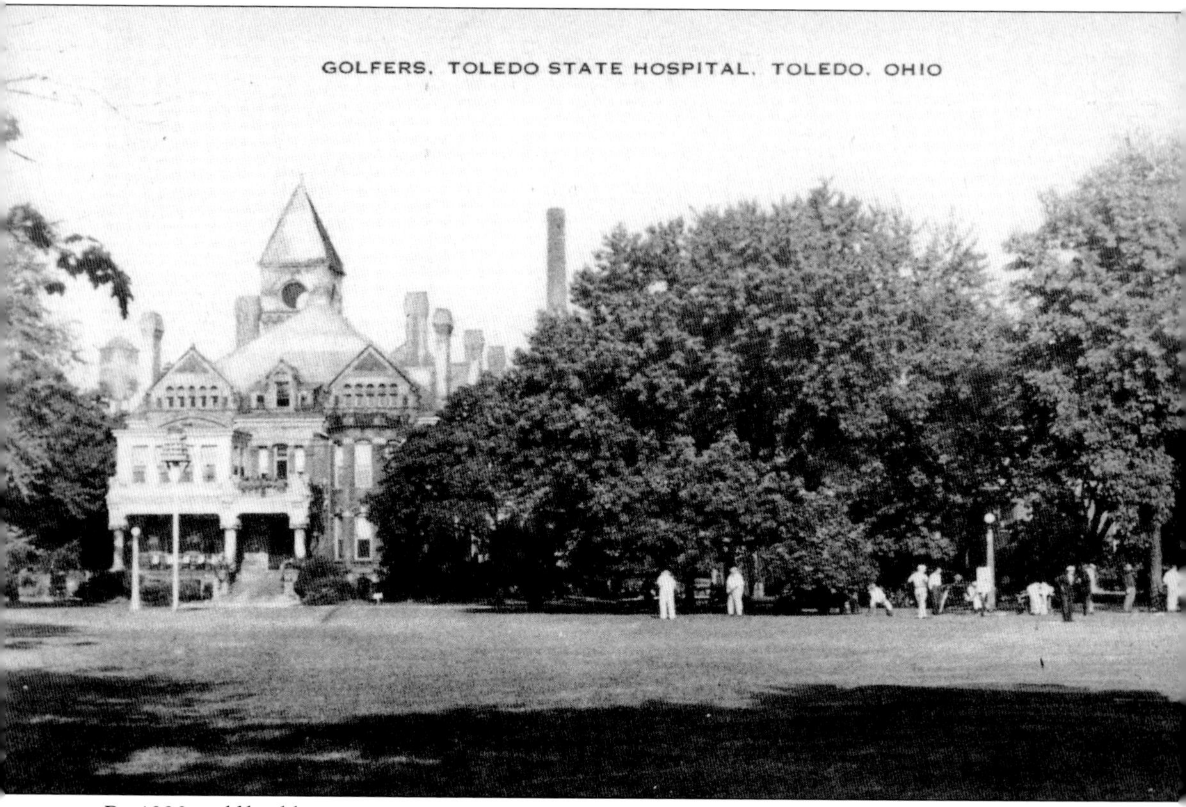

By 1930, golf had become a popular sport in the United States, and the hospital laid out a nine-hole course on the grounds for the enjoyment of the patients and staff. The course was located along the hospital's frontage on Detroit Avenue and wrapped around the corner on Arlington Avenue. Many tournaments were held on the course between patients and staff. (TLCPL.)

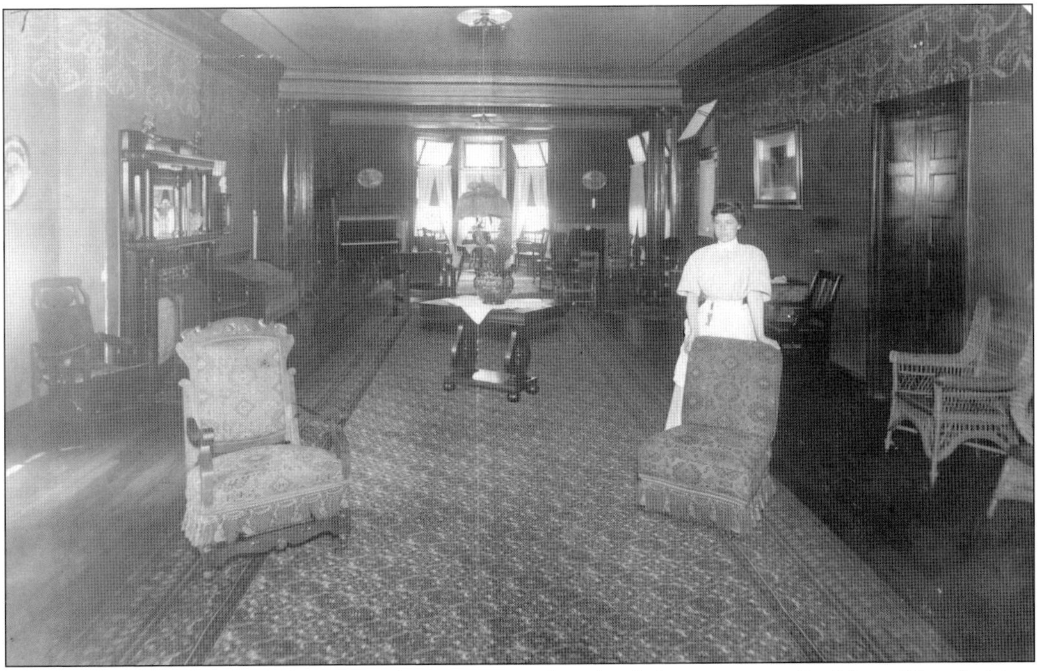

In 1928, the hospital's social services division opened in the Administration Building. This division established an outpatient clinic through which trial home visits were supervised. While the clinic was intended to serve the hospital's outpatients, members of the community were accepted as patients as well. (TLCPL.)

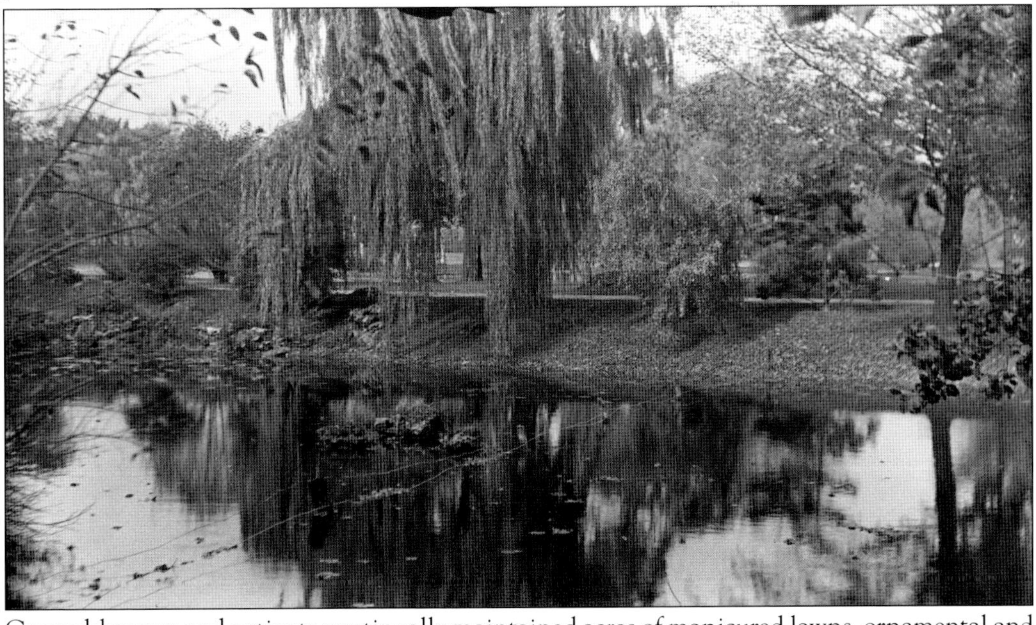

Groundskeepers and patients continually maintained acres of manicured lawns, ornamental and shade trees, shrubs, aquatic plants, and flowers during the spring, summer, and fall. They groomed the golf course; built and resurfaced miles of service roads, drives, and parking areas; and kept them in good repair. In the winter, they managed snow and ice removal and cared for mowers and other equipment. (TLCPL.)

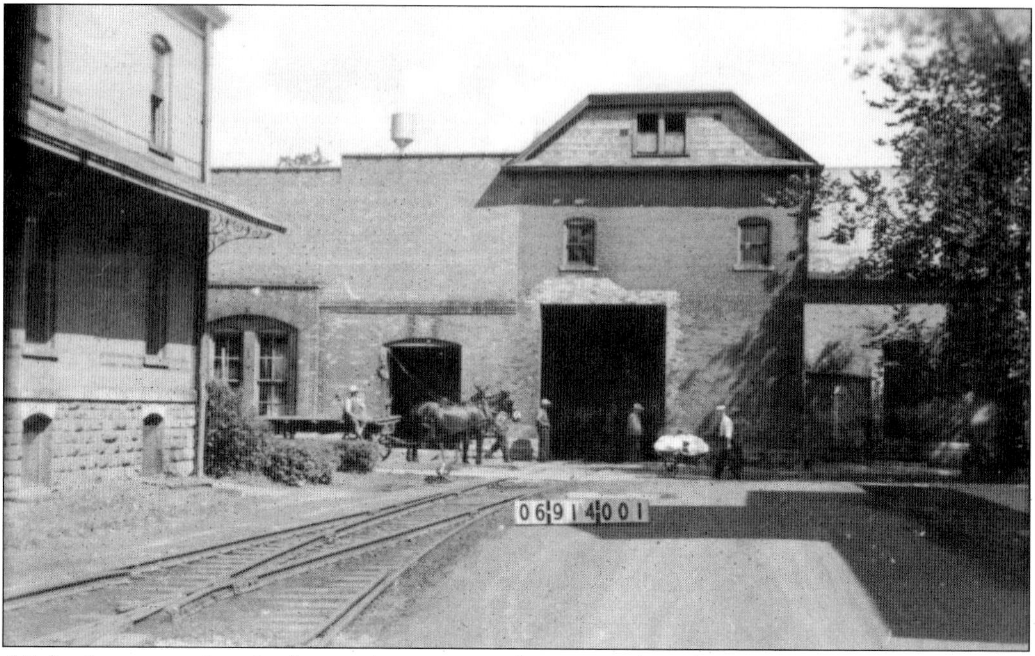

All food consumed at the hospital was received, processed, and prepared in the Food Service Building for delivery to the kitchen. Notice the horse-drawn wagon still in use. Food preparation was a huge operation at the hospital; three meals a day were served to over 2,500 patients and staff in 1930. (TLCPL.)

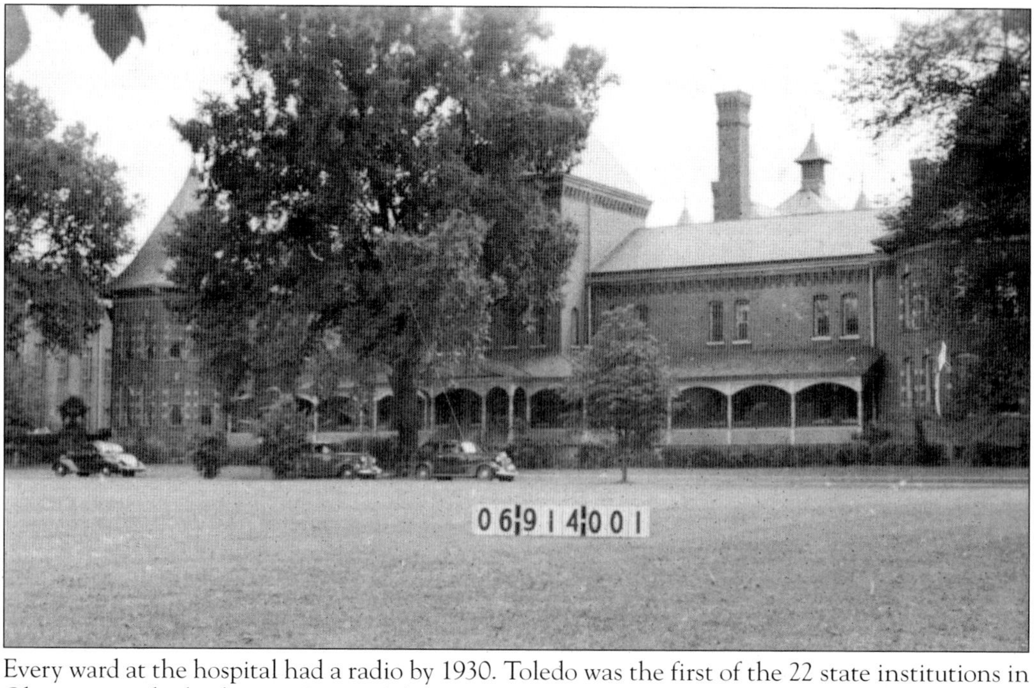

Every ward at the hospital had a radio by 1930. Toledo was the first of the 22 state institutions in Ohio to provide this luxury. Some of the sets were purchased with proceeds from the hospital gift shop, and some were donated by friends. Listening to music helped put the patients in a healthier and happier frame of mind. This c. 1937 photograph shows the Men's Hospital. (TLCPL.)

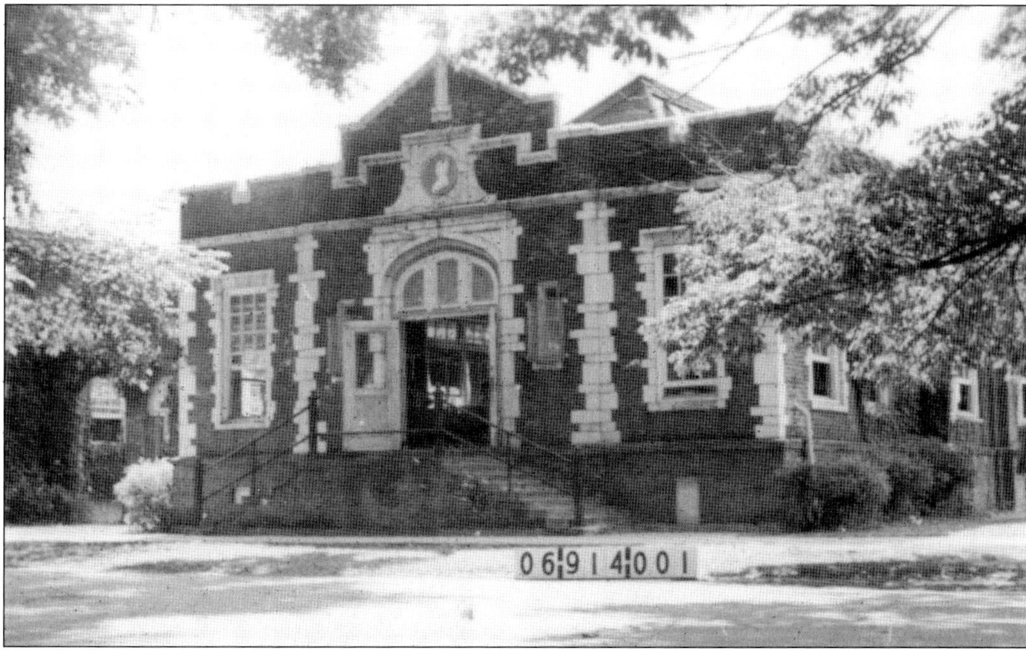

The Laundry Building was erected before 1900 and expanded in 1904. Each week, 7,000 bedsheets and more than 2,500 pillowcases were washed and ironed, along with hundreds of tablecloths, thousands of bath and kitchen towels, medical linens, and the personal laundry of 2,300 patients and 250 employees. (TLCPL.)

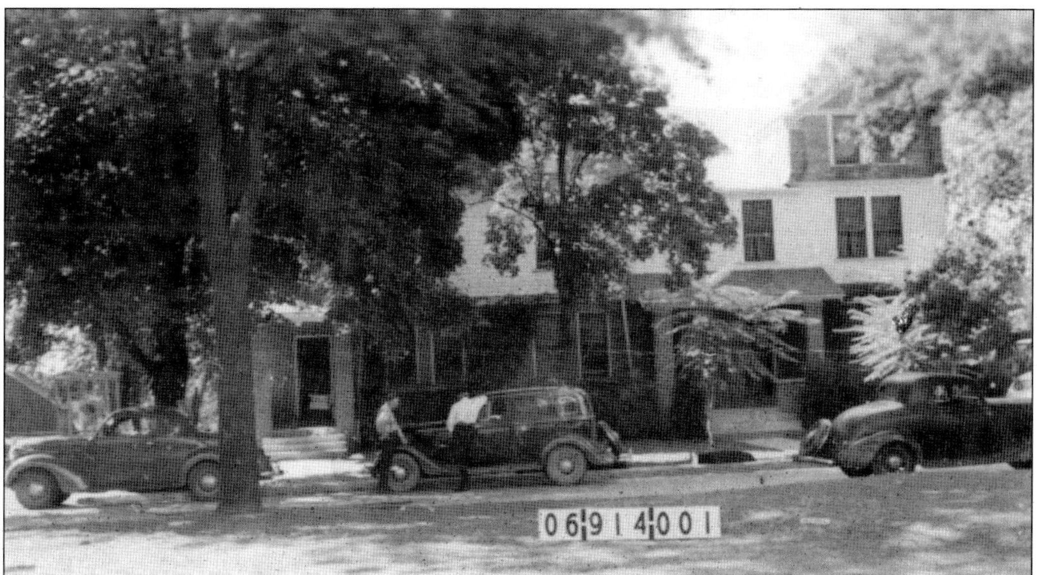

One of the staff residences, the Tri-plex, was originally a simple block building of three units. In 1900, wings were added so that each unit could have a kitchen, closet, and porch. Several other employee and physician residences were built on the grounds as well. Living on the grounds was desirable because staff had to be available in case of an emergency. (TLCPL.)

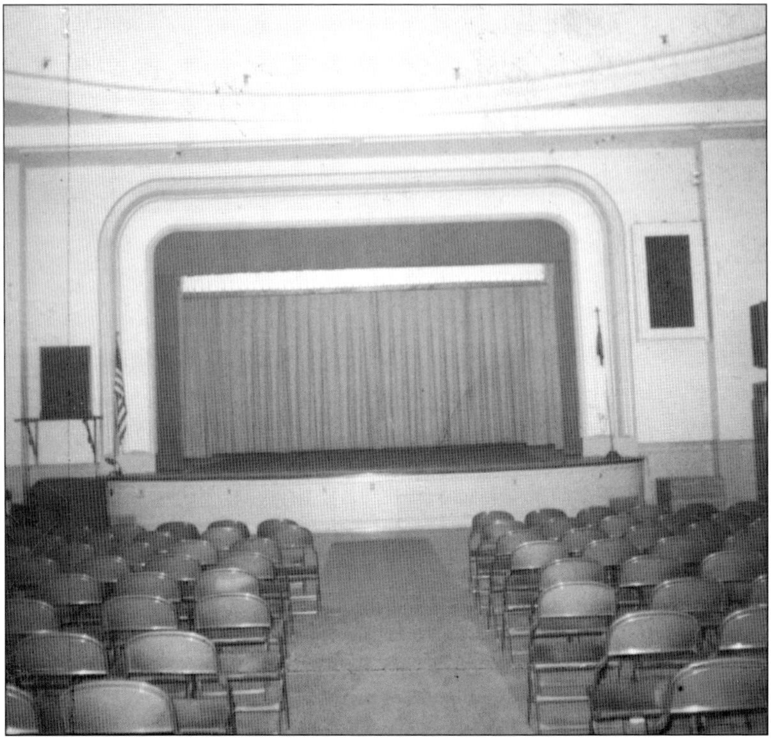

Many events designed to divert the troubled mind were held in the Entertainment Hall. In 1930, Dr. Fordyce boasted that the hospital would begin a program of "talking pictures" twice a week for patient and staff entertainment. He also reported that patients enjoyed the golf course so much that they were building a miniature golf course in the basement of one of the cottages for use during the winter. (NOPH.)

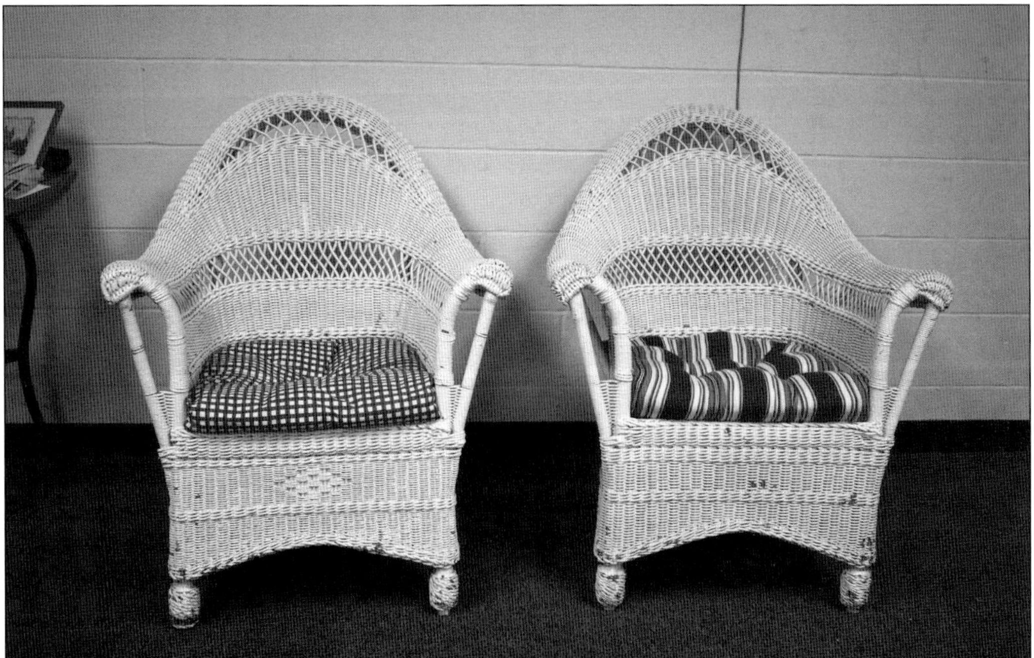

Wicker chairs like these were made by male patients during occupational therapy sessions held in the Industrial Building. The chairs were used in many of the wards and cottages and can be seen in several of the photographs in this book. Wicker chairs, along with other items of furniture made by patients, were sold in the hospital store. (Photograph by author.)

Most of the vegetables consumed at the hospital were grown on its farm. In 1930, it produced 250,000 pounds of cabbage, most of which was made into kraut and stored in the Kraut House, located across Arlington Avenue next to the Old Cemetery. Potatoes and apples were also stored in this building. (NOPH.)

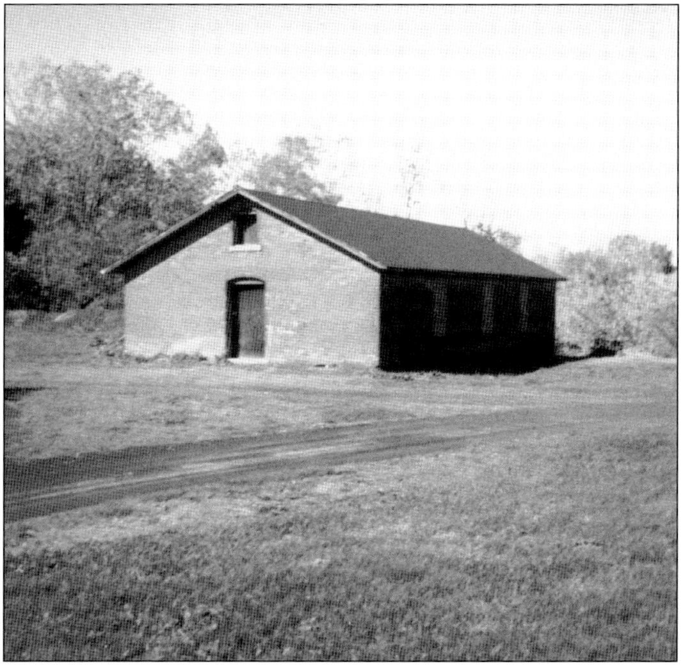

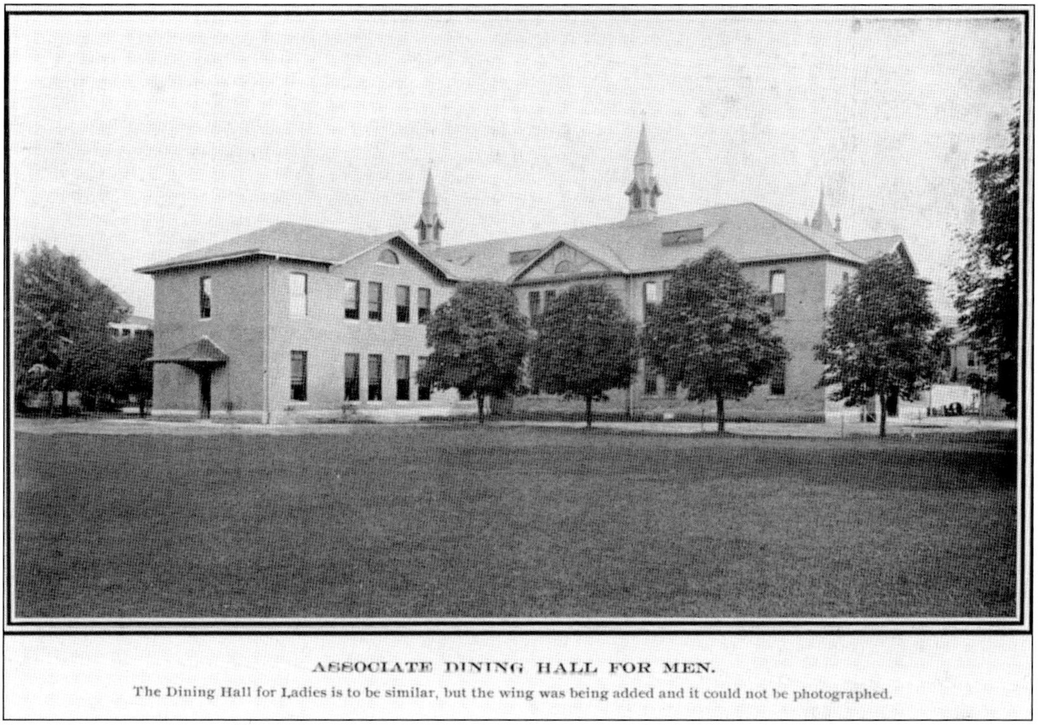
ASSOCIATE DINING HALL FOR MEN.
The Dining Hall for Ladies is to be similar, but the wing was being added and it could not be photographed.

The farm's cultivation operation thrived in the 1930s. Onions, cabbage, carrots, lettuce, corn, tomatoes, rhubarb, and pickling cucumbers were grown on the farm. There were apple and peach orchards, and raspberries, cherries, blueberries, grapes, and cantaloupe were grown. All of the fruits and vegetables produced were either served to the patients in the dining halls or canned for winter consumption. (NOPH.)

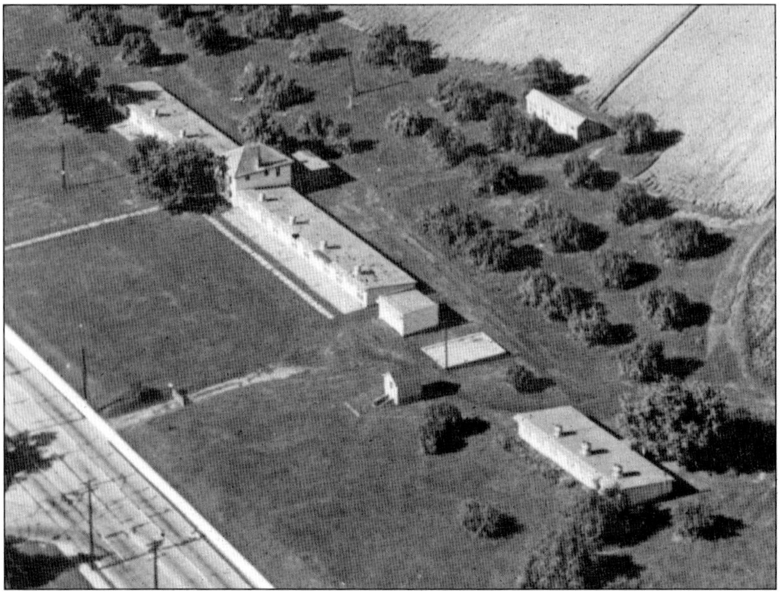

The new poultry house also opened in 1930. The poultry operation supplied the hospital with 8,000 dozen eggs per year, and with the new facility, it was forecast that production would increase to 20,000 dozen the next year. The new house was 270 feet long and could house more than 2,000 laying hens. (CC.)

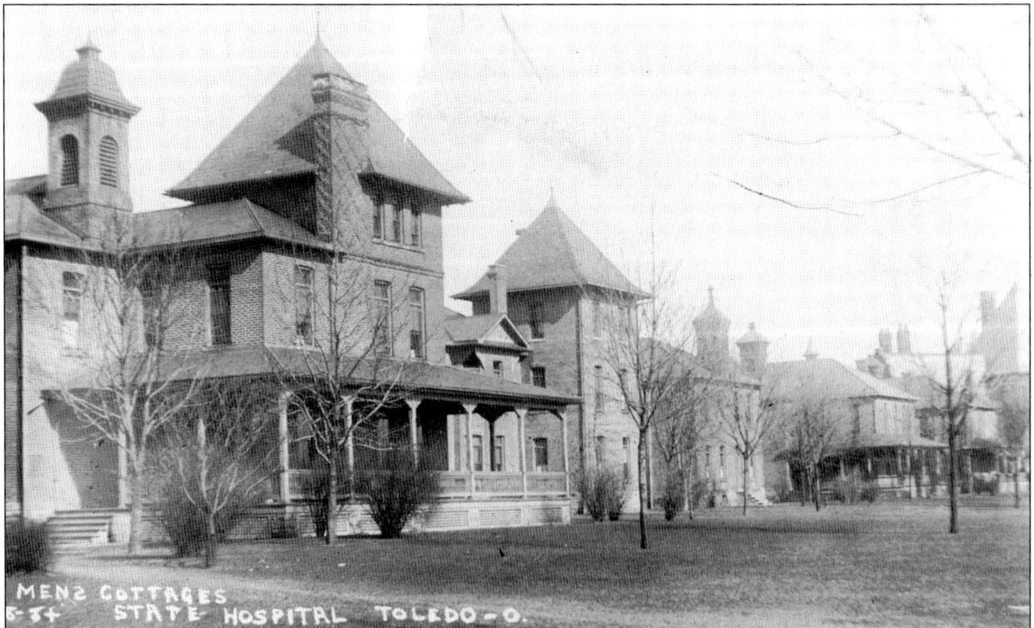

In 1933, a cafeteria for male patients was opened. Dr. Fordyce believed that the process of choosing one's own food was a "mental drill," an act of independence that helped give the patient self-confidence. He noted an improvement in manners and decorum as a result and considered the return of such behavior as a step toward the return of sanity. (TLCPL.)

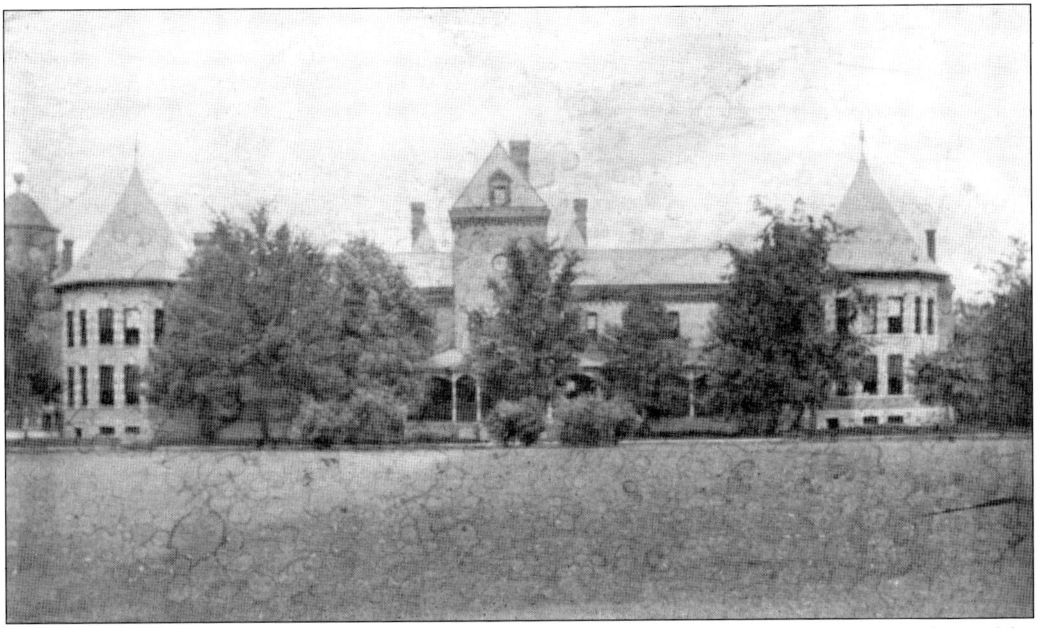

The hospital opened its metrazol clinic in 1934. Metrazol was a drug given to cause epileptic-like convulsions and was used to treat dementia praecox, now known as schizophrenia. It was difficult to administer this drug, however, because of one of its side effects—it caused feelings of terror immediately prior to the onset of the seizures—and patients feared taking it. (NOPH.)

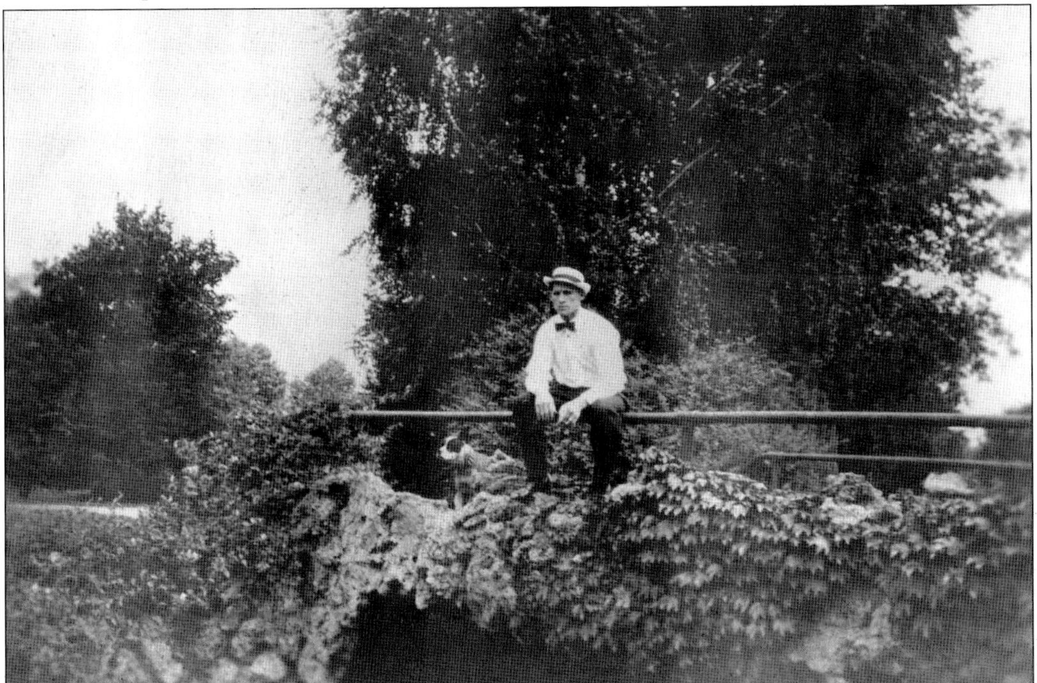

Insulin shock therapy was also used to treat dementia praecox, and the hospital opened a clinic for this treatment in 1934 as well. Insulin was injected in large doses to lower the patient's blood sugar level until coma was induced. This was done repeatedly over the course of several weeks. (TLCPL.)

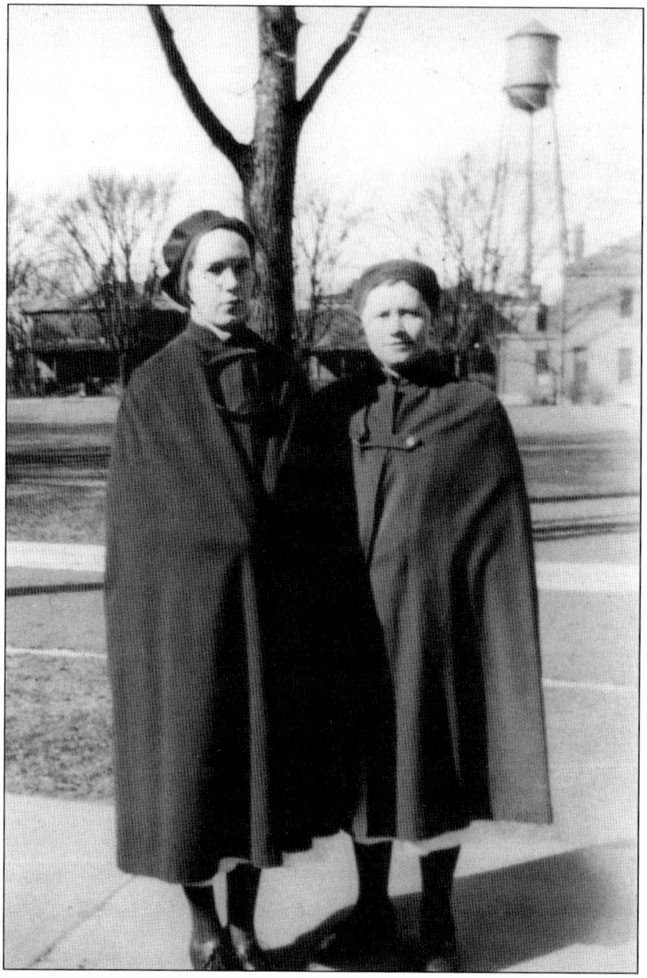

The nursing school established a three-year accredited program with a six-month specialization in psychiatry in 1933. Affiliated with the Lucas County Hospital, students attended lectures and clinicals at both hospitals, and all received general medical and psychiatric training. During World War II, the school was discontinued due to a staff shortage. (NOPH.)

The patient library was built in 1938. It was a project of the Public Works Administration, part of Pres. Franklin D. Roosevelt's New Deal, aimed at creating jobs and increasing public welfare. The hospital's portion of the cost was paid with profits from the sales of patient-made crafts in the hospital store. (NOPH.)

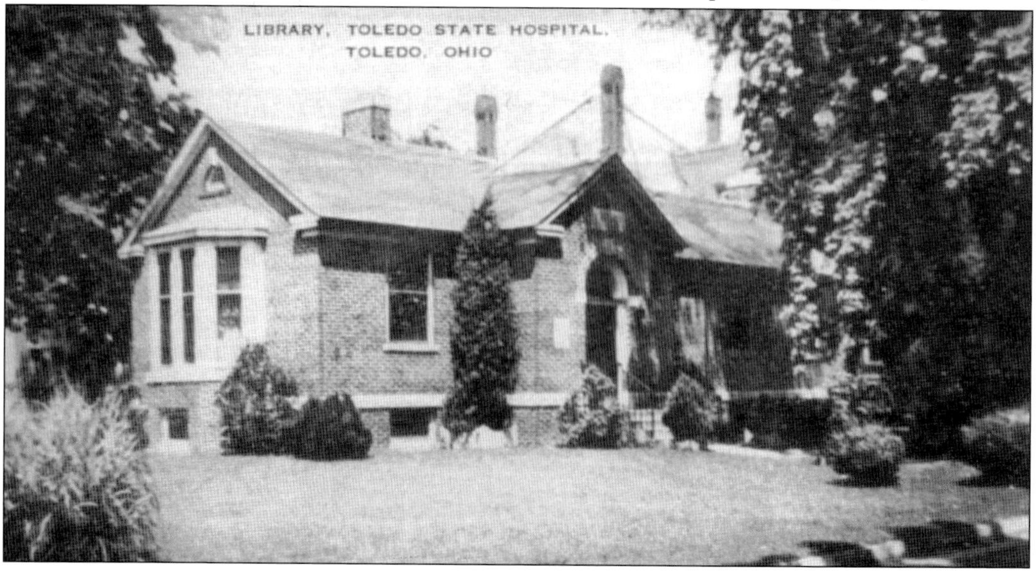

Elizabeth Ross Frank was a patient at the hospital for 46 years. She had attacked her husband with a knife, believing that he wanted to harm her. Her husband escorted her to the hospital and officially relinquished responsibility for her care in 1894. She was diagnosed with chronic mania, which her family believed was from childbirth injuries, although Elizabeth's father had suffered "dethronement of reason" and committed suicide. Two years later, Elizabeth had improved enough for a trial home visit, but her paranoia returned, and she was sent back to the hospital. Three decades later, she was again eligible for discharge, but her family chose to decline. She died there in 1940. While Elizabeth was a patient, she made the quilt pictured below—42 squares perfectly aligned and painstakingly hand-stitched. (Right, Joanne Passet; below, photograph by author.)

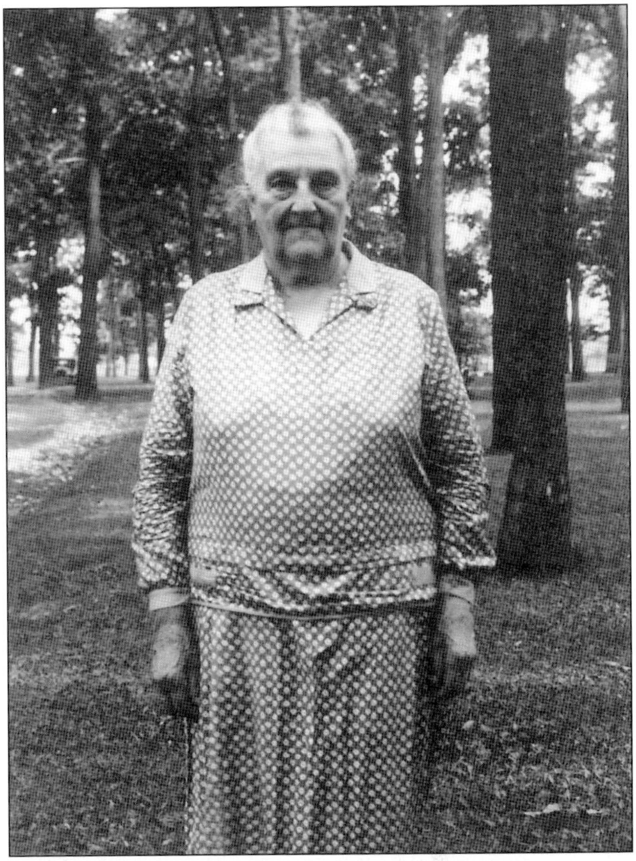

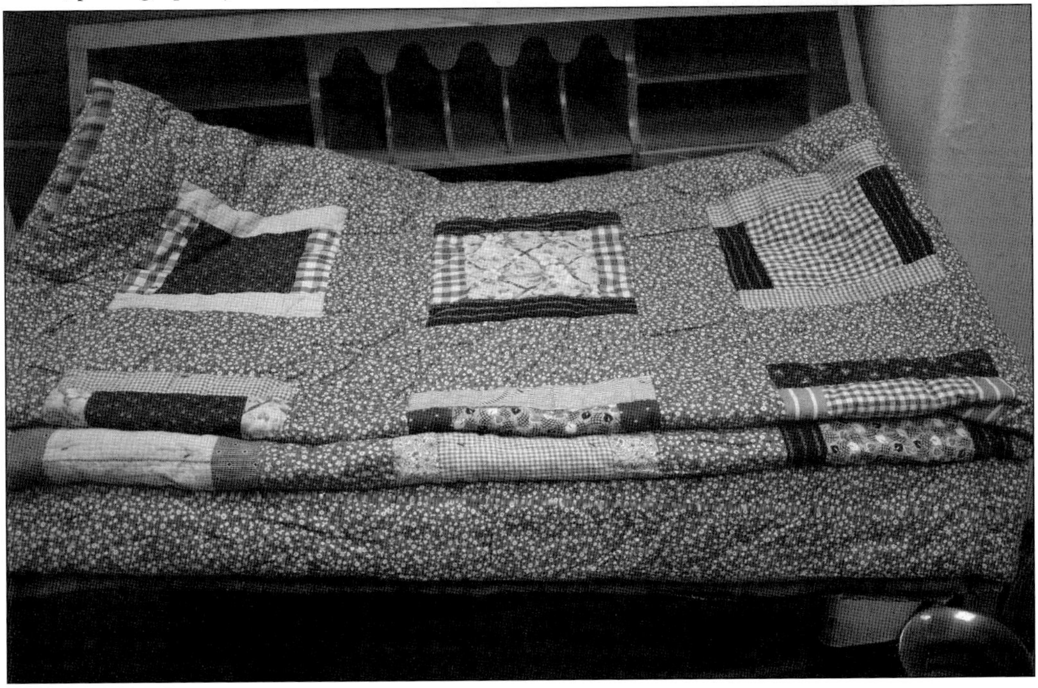

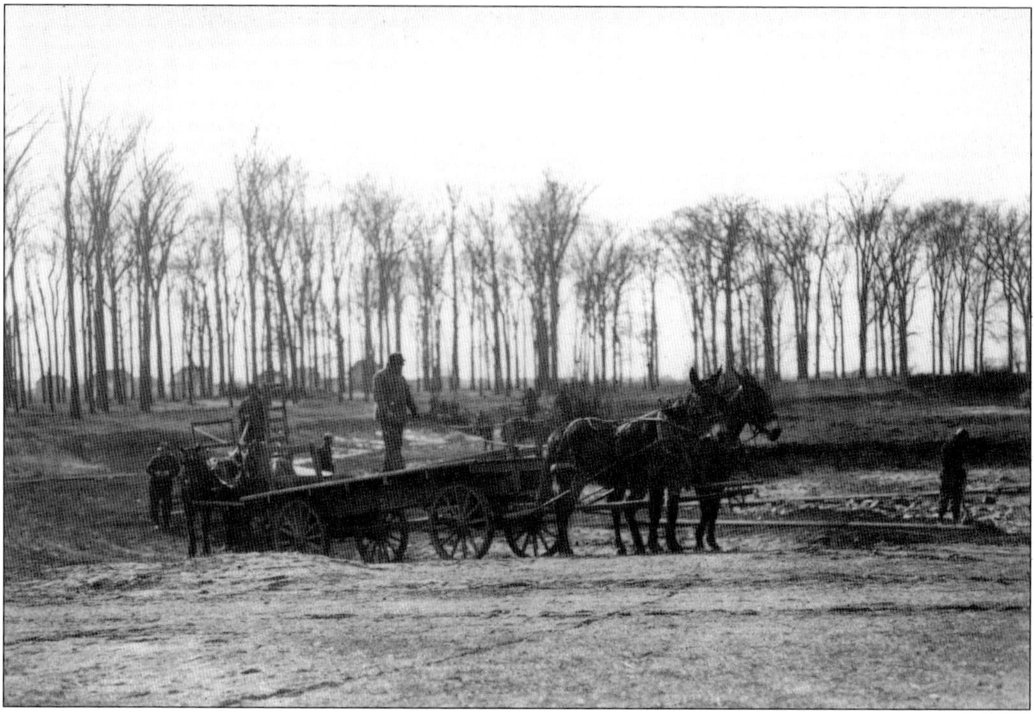

Workers used mules and carts to fill in the large lake formerly known as the Sunken Garden. The lake had provided a great deal of beauty to the grounds, and served as a spot for recreational activities and a source of ice in the winter. However, it was so shallow that it tended to transform into a mud hole during dry weather. (NOPH.)

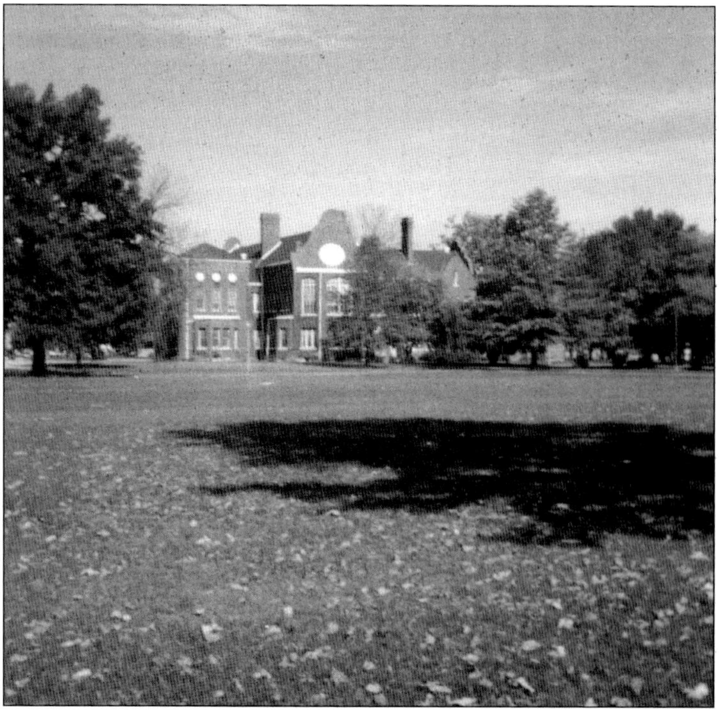

The Sunken Garden was filled in 1937. Because it was so shallow, it had become a chronic problem, often drying up to nothing but mud or a stagnant pond and breeding ground for mosquitos. The absence of the lake vastly altered this previously picturesque view of the Women's Hospital. (NOPH.)

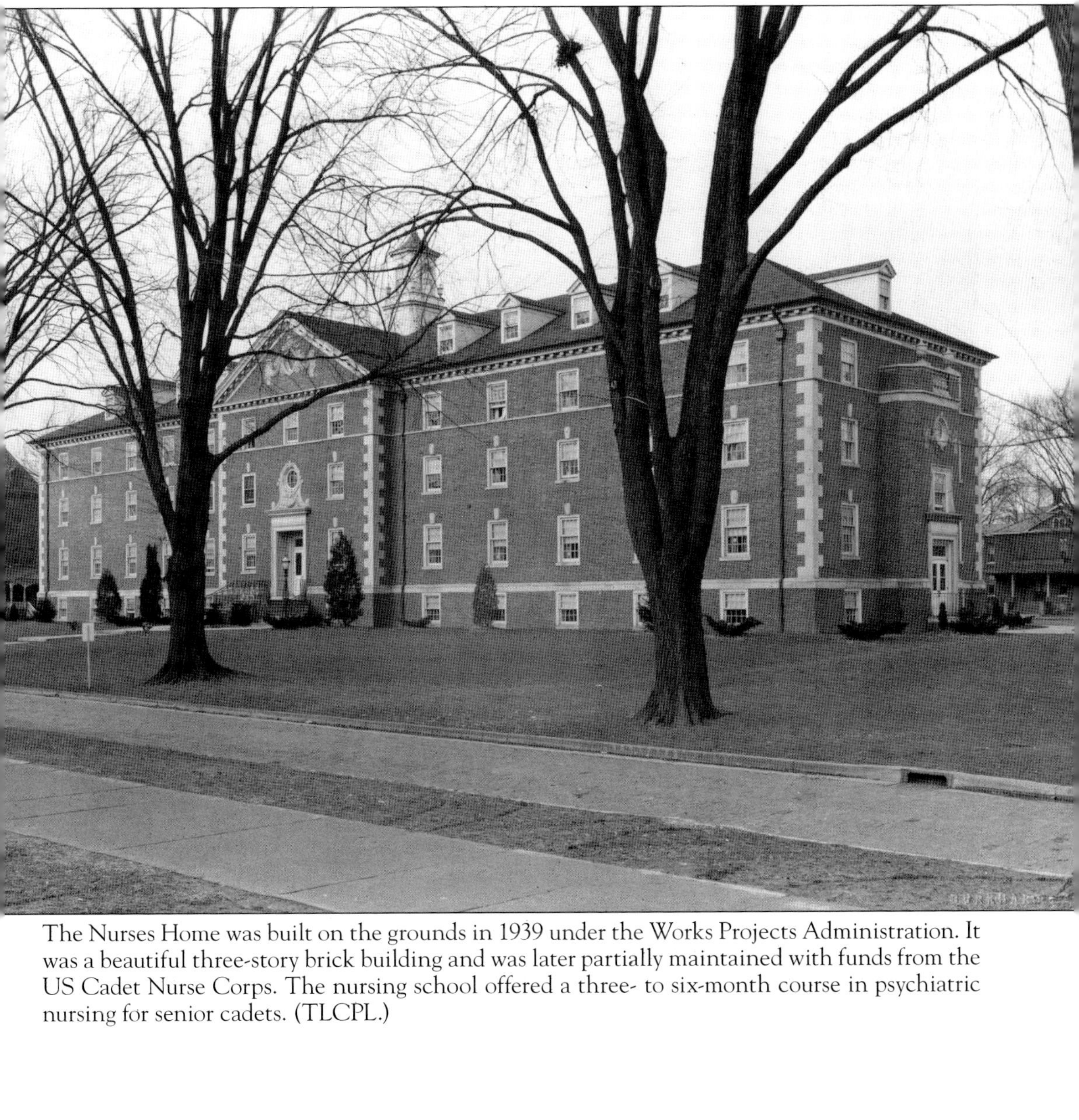

The Nurses Home was built on the grounds in 1939 under the Works Projects Administration. It was a beautiful three-story brick building and was later partially maintained with funds from the US Cadet Nurse Corps. The nursing school offered a three- to six-month course in psychiatric nursing for senior cadets. (TLCPL.)

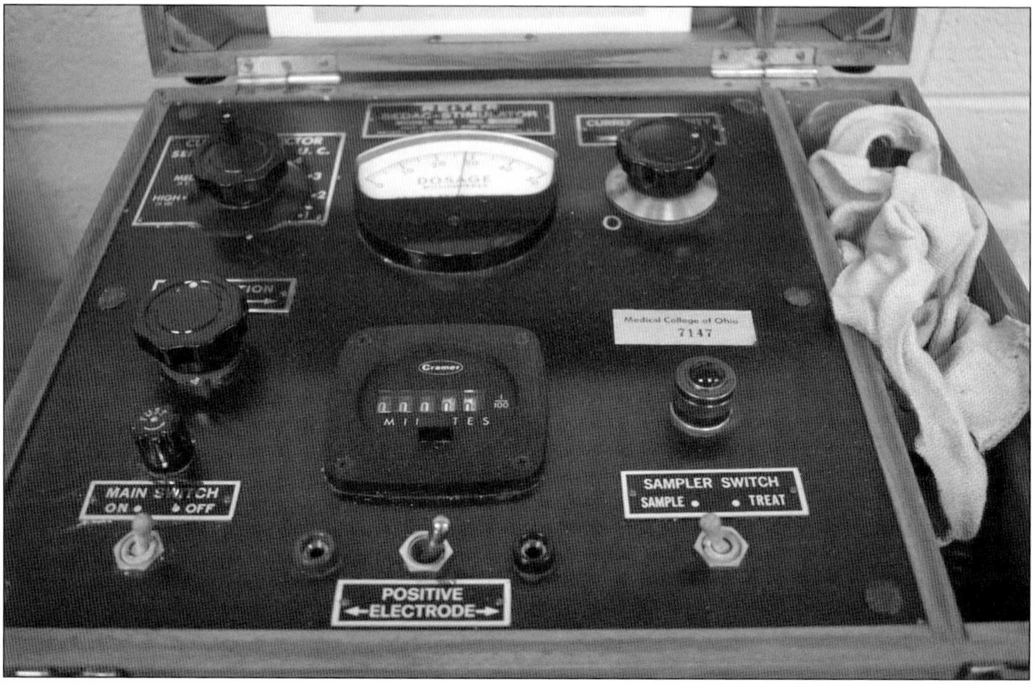

Electroconvulsive shock therapy was first introduced at the hospital in 1941. Electricity was administered to patients to produce seizures, which often eased their symptoms. It was particularly effective in treating depression and was used as an alternative to metrazol therapy, which caused feelings of terror immediately prior to the seizure. Unfortunately, it was also sometimes used to control unruly patients. (Photograph by author.)

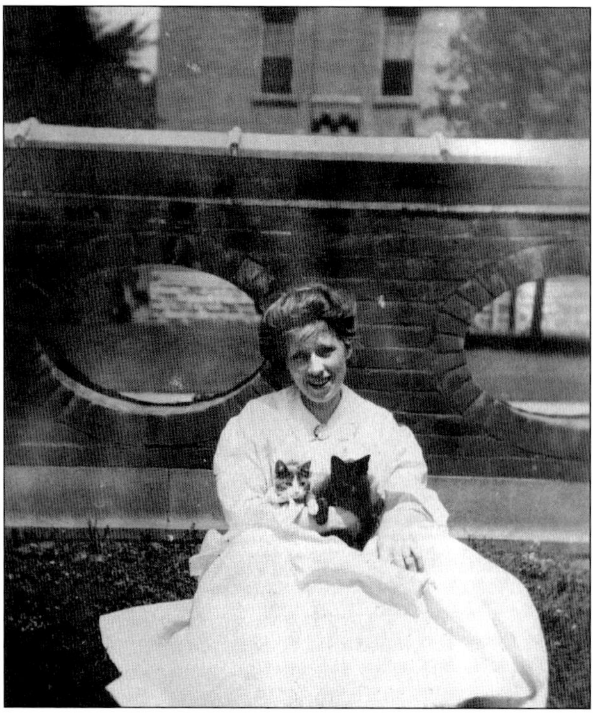

Use of the psychosurgery lobotomy began in the early 1940s. It was a procedure in which the neurological connections in the front of the brain were severed. The goal was to reduce the symptoms of many kinds of mental disorders, but the operation frequently caused other serious impairments and side effects. Lobotomies were rarely performed at the Toledo State Hospital. (TLCPL.)

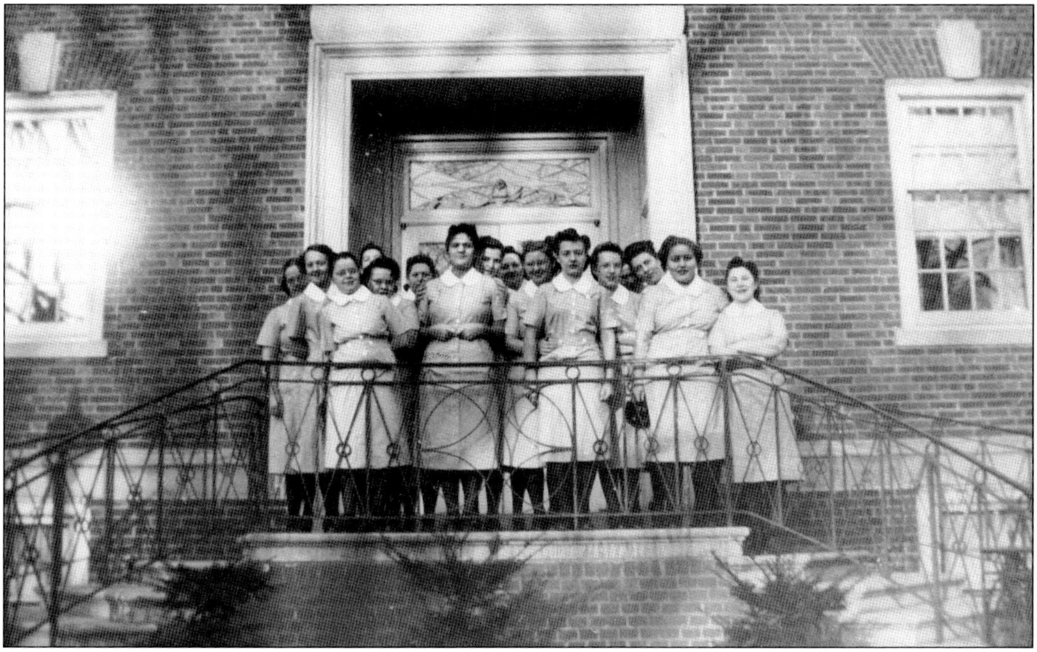

A class of nursing students poses on the steps of the Nurses Home in 1941. As World War II began, the hospital's nursing staff decreased as many joined the military and went overseas, and the nursing school was forced to close. At the same time, war-related stress, both in returning soldiers and civilians at home, resulted in an increase in admissions, and the hospital's population swelled once again. (NOPH.)

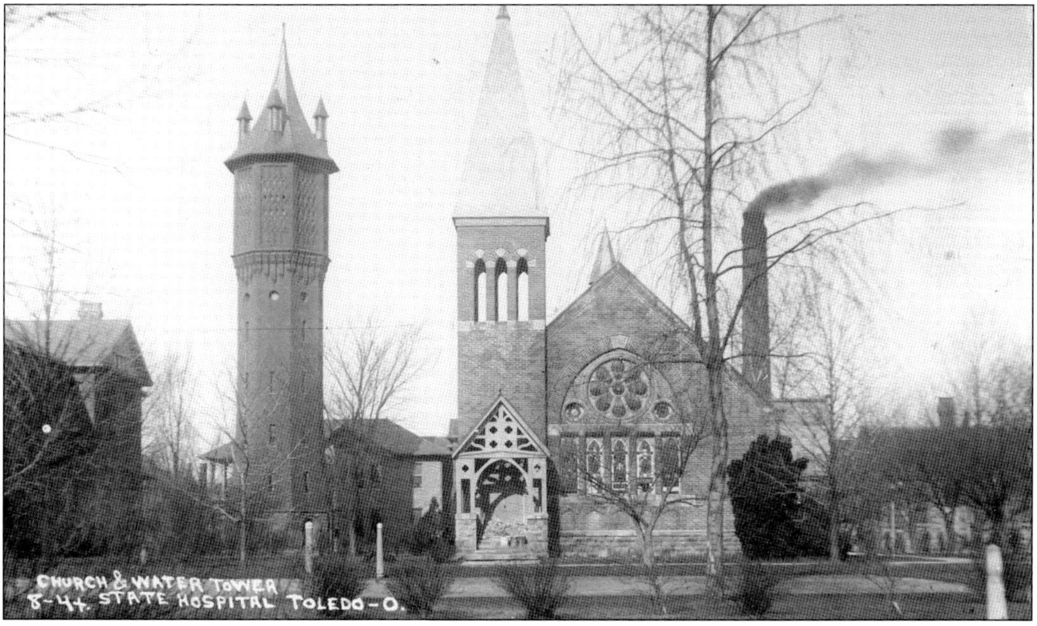

In 1943, the chapel was dedicated to serving the hospital's Catholic population exclusively and was officially named St. Dymphna Chapel after the patron saint of those suffering from mental illness. Protestant services were also held in the building until the 1920s, when the congregation became too large, and services were moved to the Entertainment Hall. (NOPH.)

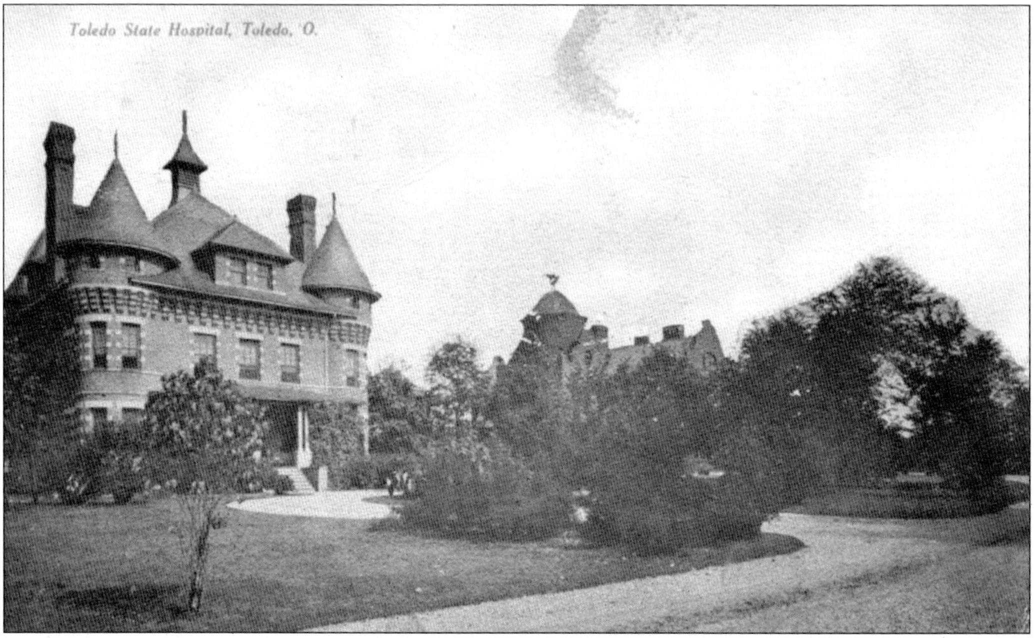

By 1944, the hospital had 425 employees, including eight doctors, two social workers, and two chaplains—one Catholic and one Protestant. In addition to holding religious services, the chaplains visited patients in the hospitals and cottages and provided personal and religious counseling to patients as part of their therapy. (NOPH.)

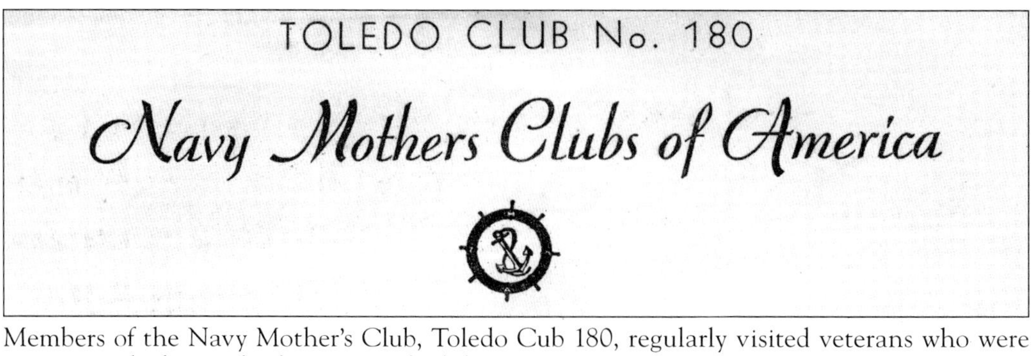
TOLEDO CLUB No. 180

Navy Mothers Clubs of America

Members of the Navy Mother's Club, Toledo Cub 180, regularly visited veterans who were patients at the hospital. The veterans had their own cottage, Cottage 2, and the club's members held monthly parties and dances for them there for 16 years. (Center for Archival Collections, Bowling Green State University.)

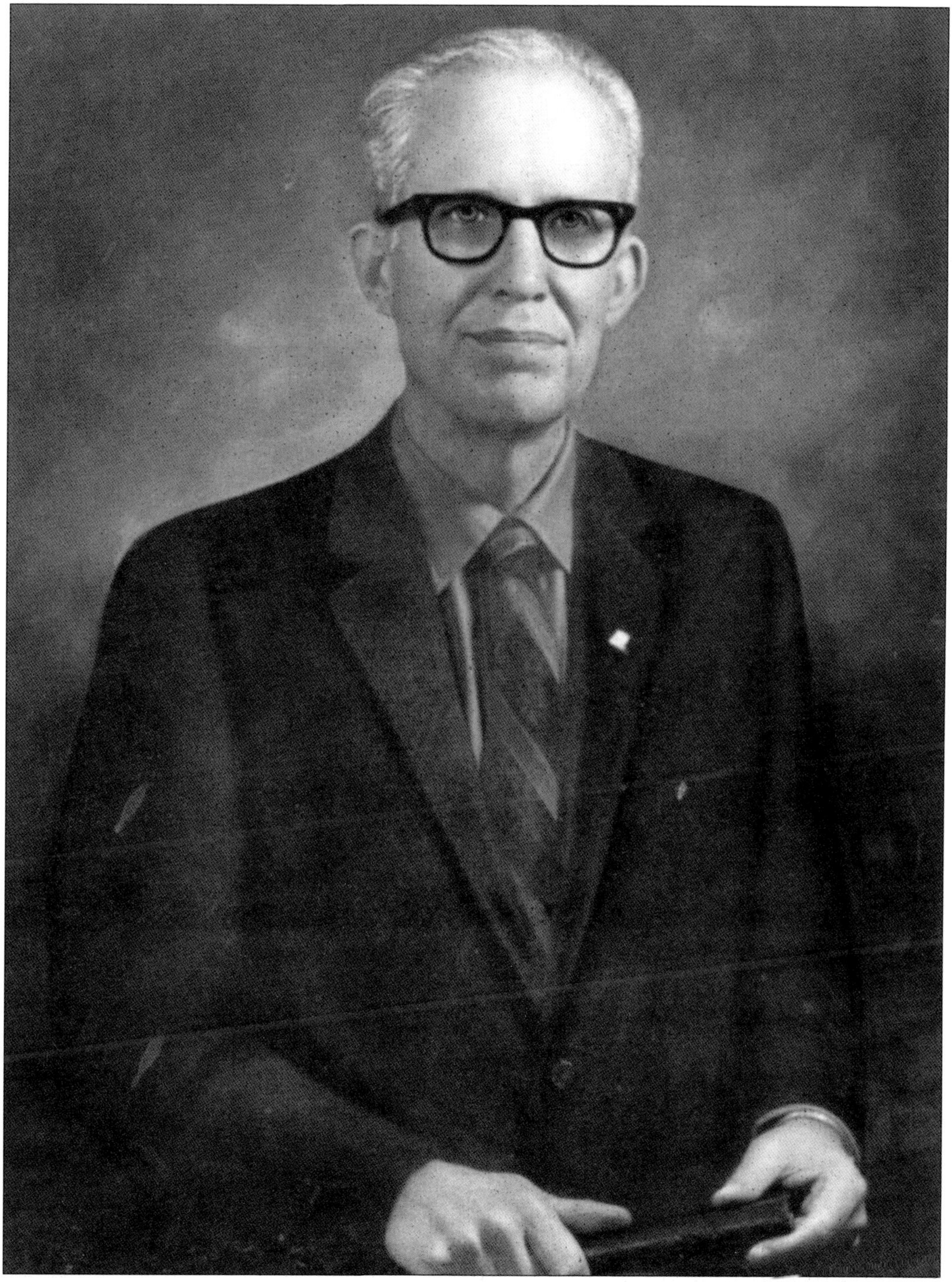

In 1946, Dr. Joseph E. Duty succeeded Dr. Fordyce as superintendent. He would serve the hospital until 1968. During his tenure, he faced a physically crumbling and overcrowded hospital and witnessed vast improvements in medications and the effect they had on his patients. He was known for his advocacy for improved facilities for the mentally ill and educating the public to dispel stigma. (NOPH.)

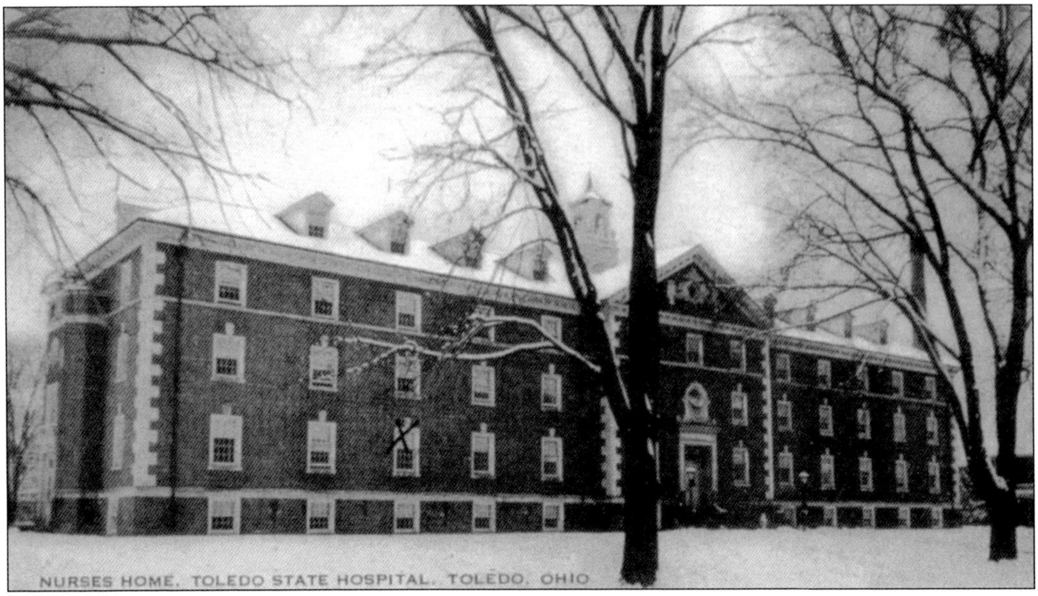

A survey conducted in 1948 by volunteers for the Ohio Citizens Council reported a need for an increase in salaries for nurses, job classification, more nurses with psychiatric training, and more opportunities for continuing education. Similar needs were reported for attendants, with the additional need for better living quarters with adequate facilities. (NOPH.)

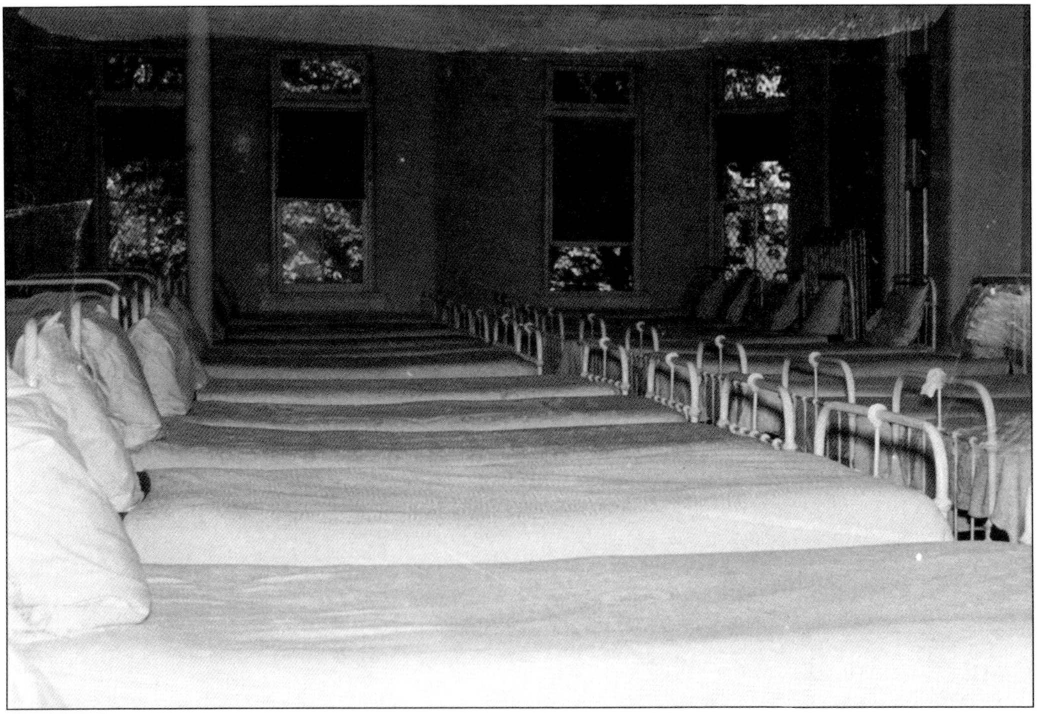

In 1948, the hospital's patient-to-doctor ratio was 275:1. The standard set by the American Psychiatric Association for an institution the size of Toledo State Hospital was 31:1. Although few hospitals were able to meet the APA's standards, Toledo's need for more doctors was desperate. The men's wards were so crowded that patients had to climb over others' beds to reach their own. (NOPH.)

Four

Plot Plans

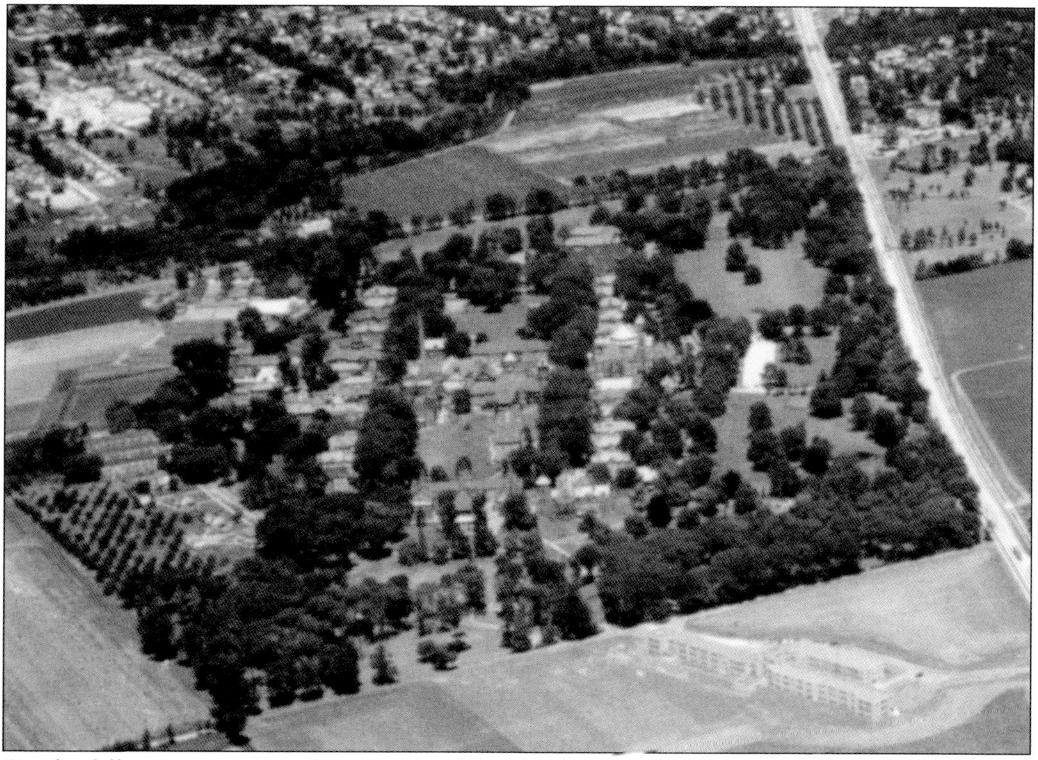

On the following pages are plot plans (and their key) for the Toledo State Hospital grounds and facilities that were drawn in 1962 as part of the Ohio Department of Finance's capital inventory project. The inventory also included floor plans of the buildings on the property, along with additional information on each building's size, use, and value. (TLCPL.)

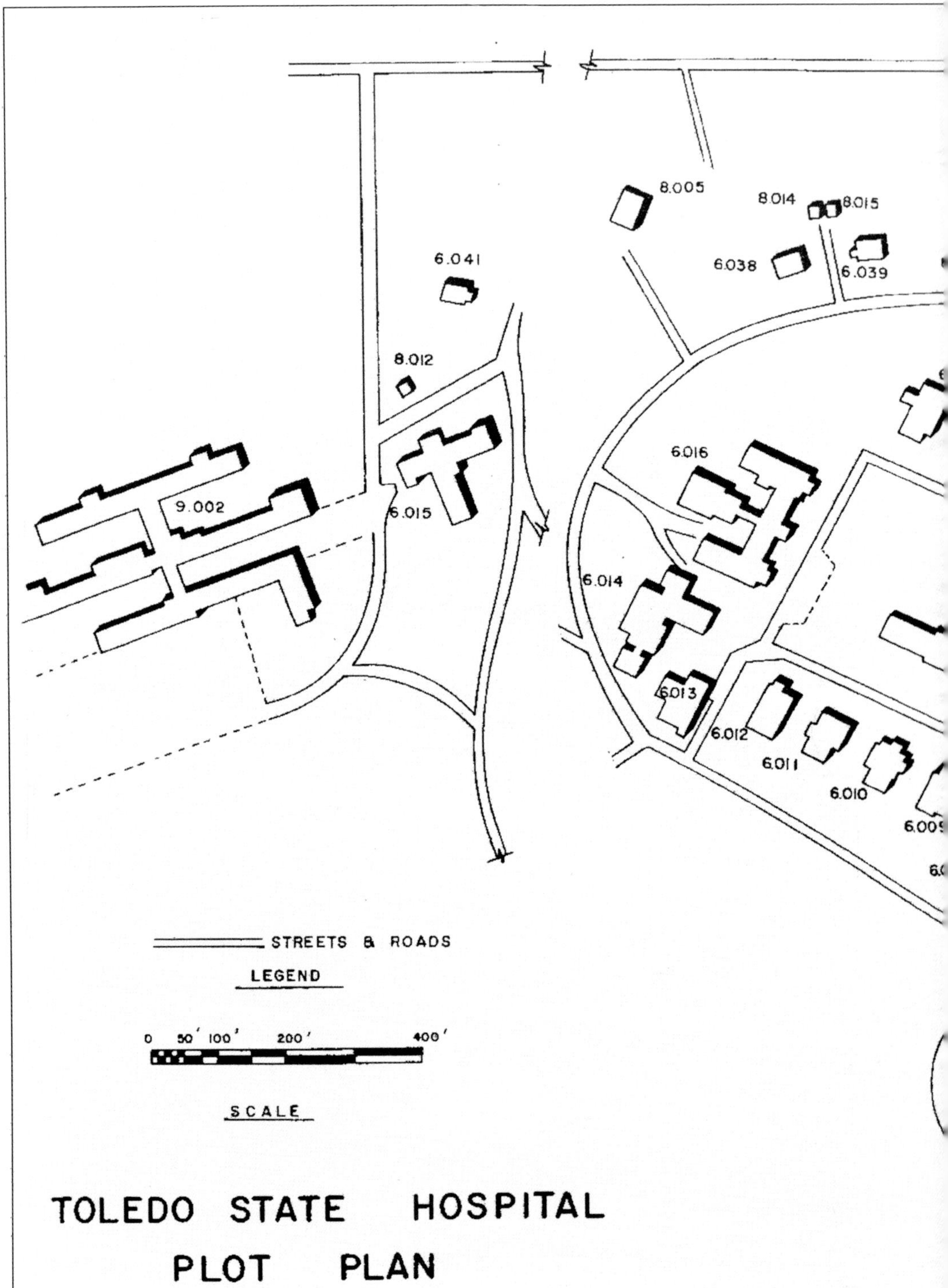

In this plan of the hospital, Arlington Avenue is along the far right, and Detroit Avenue is along the bottom. The oval drive at the bottom was the hospital's main entrance. The building

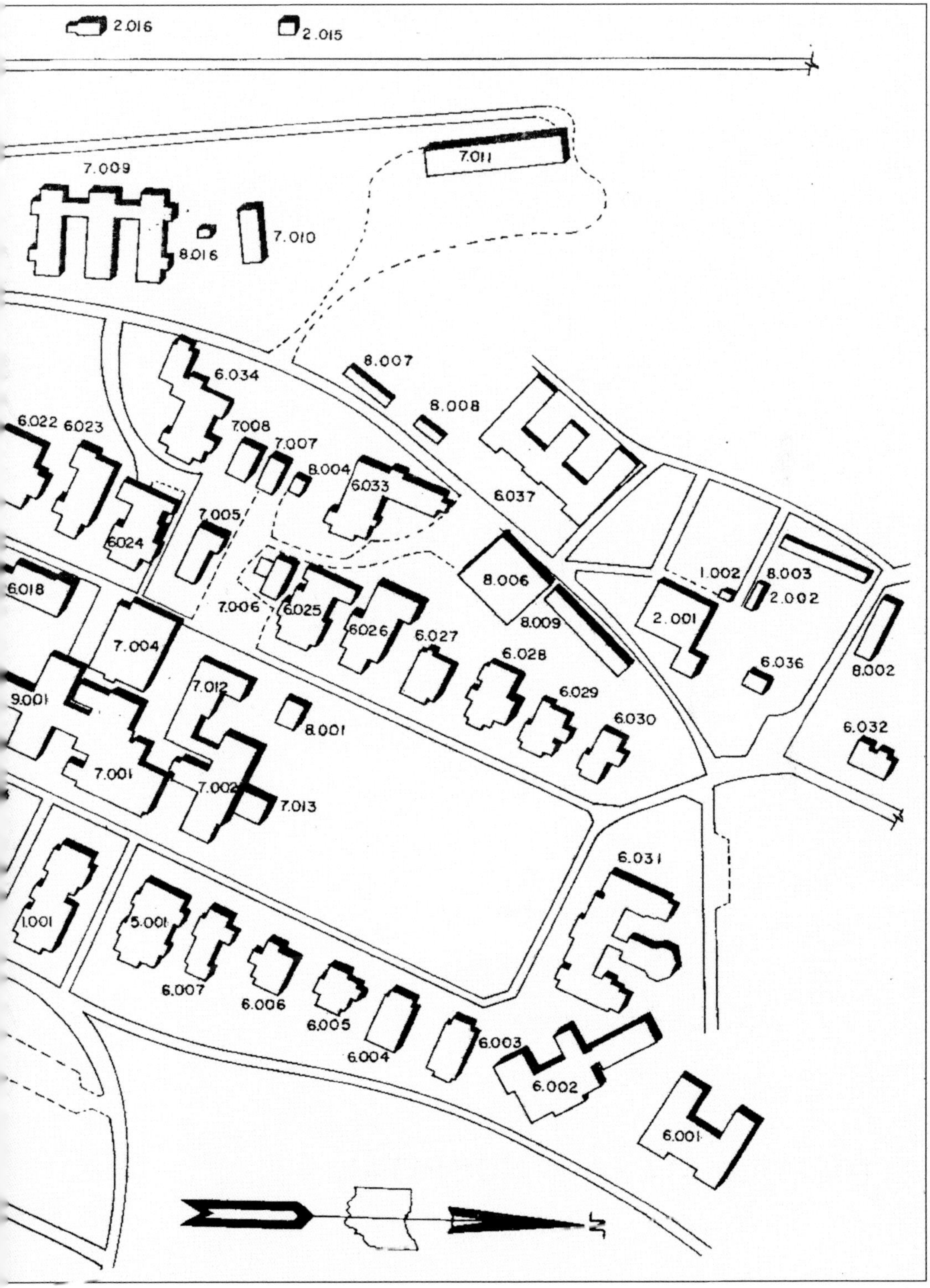

numbers correspond to the numbers in the key on pages 72 and 73. This plan was part of the Ohio Department of Finance's capital inventory conducted in 1962. (NOPH.)

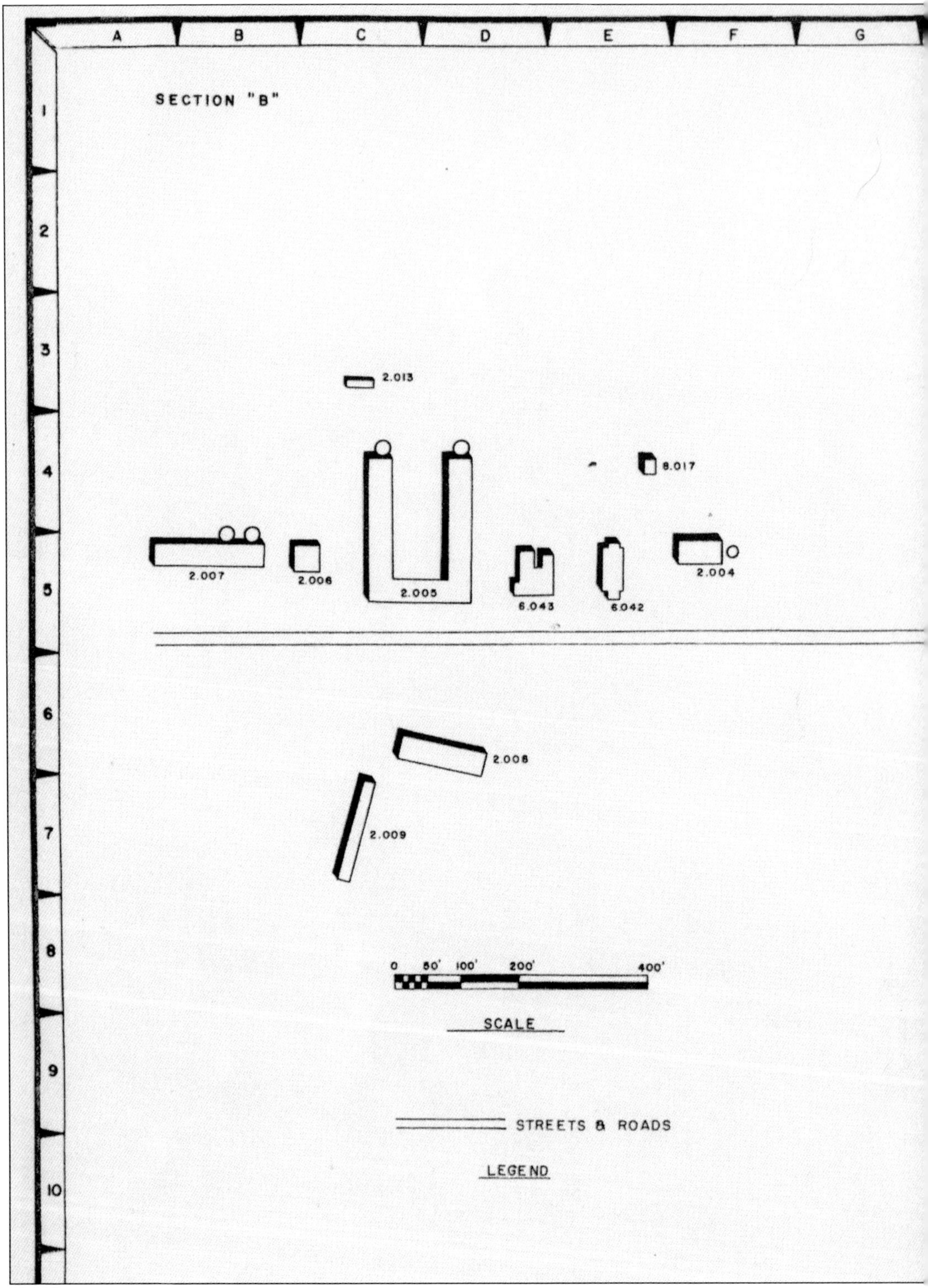

This plan shows the structures on the north side of Arlington Avenue, and two buildings on the south side of the street not pictured in the plan on the previous page. Again, the building

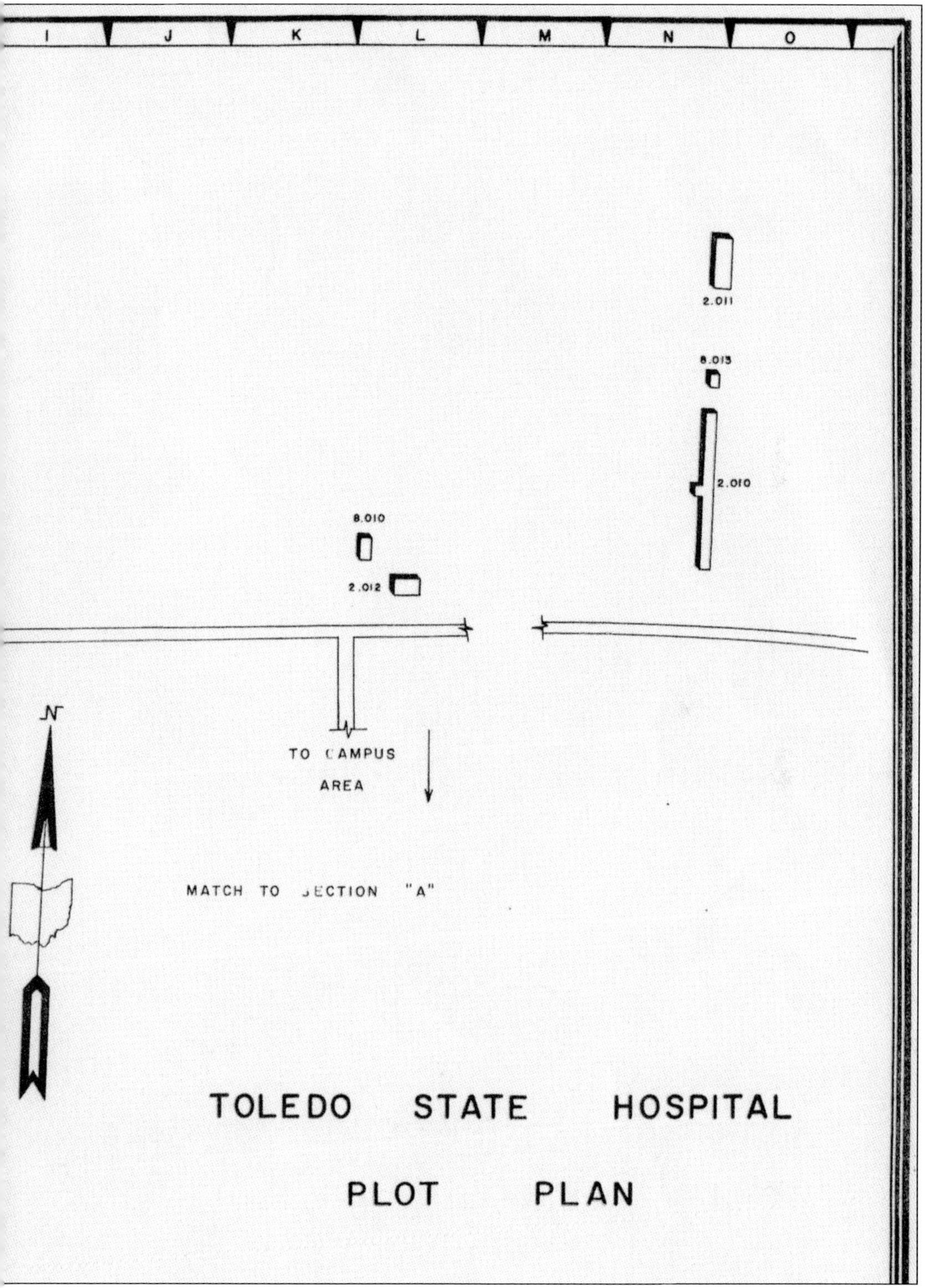

numbers correspond to the numbers in the key on pages 72 and 73, and it is also from the Ohio Department of Finance's capital inventory conducted in 1962. (NOPH.)

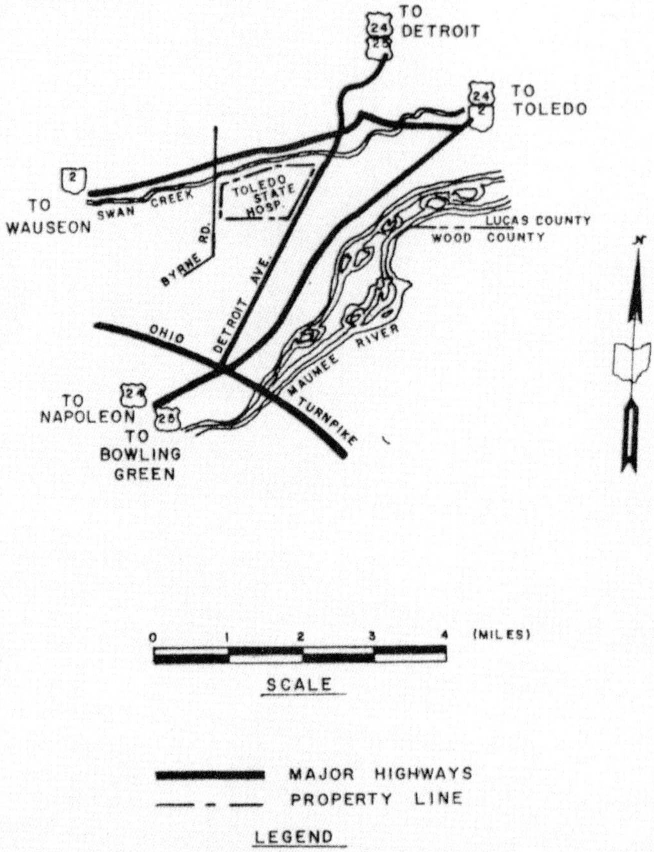

PAGE NO.	CODE NO.
287	1.001
288	1.002
289	2.001
290	2.002
290	2.003
291	2.004
292	2.005
293	2.006
294	2.007
295	2.008
296	2.009
296	2.010
297	2.011
298	2.012
298	2.013
299	2.014
299	2.015
299	2.016
300	5.001
301	5.002
302	5.003
303	6.001
304	6.002
305	6.003
306	6.004
307	6.005
308	6.006
309	6.007
310	6.008
311	6.009
312	6.010
313	6.011
314	6.012
315	6.013
316	6.014
317	6.015
318	6.016
319	6.017
320	6.018
321	6.019
322	6.020
323	6.021
324	6.022
325	6.023
326	6.024
327	6.025

TOLEDO STATE HOSPITAL

PLOT PLAN LEGEND

368

This document is the key to the building numbers on the plot plans of the hospital drawn as part of the Ohio Department of Finance's capital inventory and pictured on pages 68–71. It also shows

G NAME	INDEX NO.
ATION BUILDING	8-I
FICE	5-N
SE	6-N
RAGE	5-O
	4-H--B
BARN	5-F-B
RN	5-C-B
RN	5-B-B
RN	5-B-B
RN	6-D-B
SHED	7-C-B
BUILDING	4-N-B
HOUSE	2-J-B
ARN	5-L-B
RN	3-C-B
DING	5-H-B
LDING	1-K
LDING	1-J
T HALL	8-J
	8-H
	7-I
TTAGE	10-N
TTAGE	9-M
5	9-L
4	9-L
3	9-K
2	8-K
1	8-J
A	7-H
B	7-H
C	7-G
D	6-G
E	6-F
COTTAGE	6-F
"	5-F
"	4-D
L	5-F
HOME	6-H
AL BUILDING	5-I
K	4-H
J	4-H
H	4-I
G	4-I
F	5-J
O	5-J
12	6-K

PAGE NO.	CODE NO.	BUILDING NAME	INDEX NO.
328	6.026	COTTAGE 6	6-L
329	6.027	COTTAGE 7	6-L
330	6.028	COTTAGE 8	6-M
331	6.029	COTTAGE 9	6-M
332	6.030	COTTAGE 10	7-N
333	6.031	M BUILDING	8-N
334	6.032	TRIPLEX RESIDENCE	7-O
335	6.033	COTTAGE N	5-L
336	6.034	COTTAGE N-2	4-J
337	6.035	RESIDENCE	3-I
338	6.036	BIGELOW COTTAGE	6-O
339	6.037	COTTAGE 14	4-M
340	6.038	DOUBLE RESIDENCE	3-G
341	6.039	RESIDENCE	3-G
342	6.040	RESIDENCE	3-H
343	6.041	RESIDENCE	3-D
344	6.042	FARM COLONY BUILDING	5-E-B
345	6.043	DAIRY RESIDENCE	5-D-B
346	7.001	FOOD SERVICE COMPLEX	7-J
347	7.002	MALE HALL	7-J
348	7.003	POST OFFICE	6-L
349	7.004	OLD POWERHOUSE	6-J
350	7.005	CARPENTER SHOP	5-J
350	7.006	MASONRY SHOP	5-K
351	7.007	MORGUE	4-K
352	7.008	MACHINE SHOP	4-K
353	7.009	LAUNDRY BUILDING	2-J
354	7.010	HEATING PLANT	3-K
355	7.011	MAINTENANCE BUILDING	2-M
356	7.012	NEW FOOD SERVICE	6-J
357	7.013	COMMISSARY	7-K
358	8.001	FIRE HALL	6-K
359	8.002	GARAGE	6-O
359	8.003	"	5-O
360	8.004	POTATO HOUSE	5-K
361	8.005	OLD ICEHOUSE	2-F
362	8.006	NEW STORES BUILDING	5-M
363	8.007	GARAGE	4-L
363	8.008	"	4-L
364	8.009	"	6-M
364	8.010	OLD KRAUT HOUSE	5-L-B
365	8.011, .012	GARAGES	2-H, 4-D
365	8.013, .014	GARAGES	3-C-B, 2-G
365	8.015, .016	GARAGES	3-G, 3-J
365	8.017	GARAGE	4-E-B
366	9.001	THERAPY BUILDING	6-I
367-368	9.002	RECEIVING HOSPITAL	5-B

where the hospital was situated in northwest Ohio. (NOPH.)

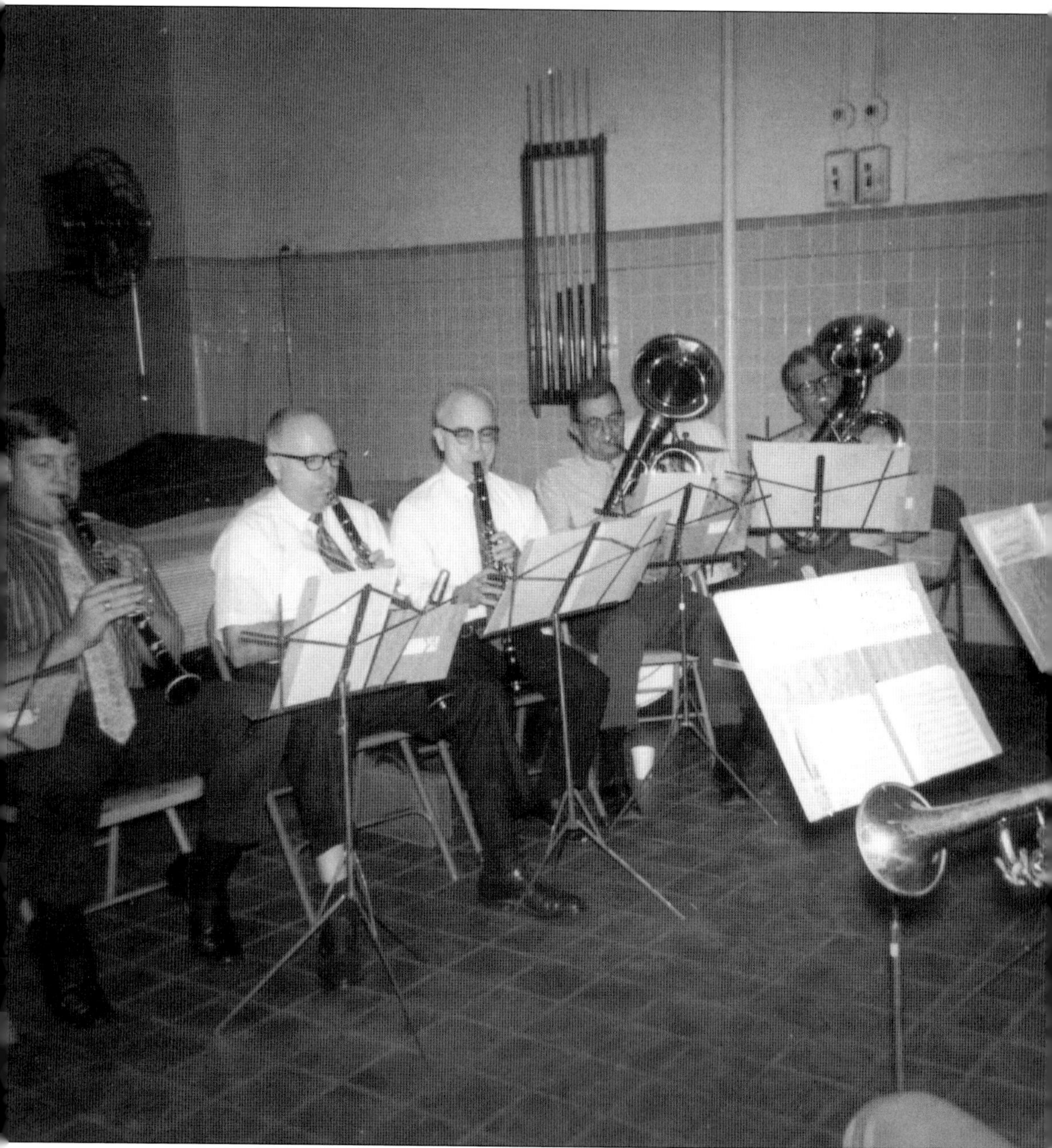

A small orchestra band is shown here providing entertainment at an unidentified hospital event around 1950. Music was always an important part of recreation and therapy at the hospital. One of the first forms of entertainment mentioned by Dr. Tobey was the hospital's cornet band, and a brass band can be seen in a photograph of one of the early baseball games on the grounds. (NOPH.)

Five

1950–1980

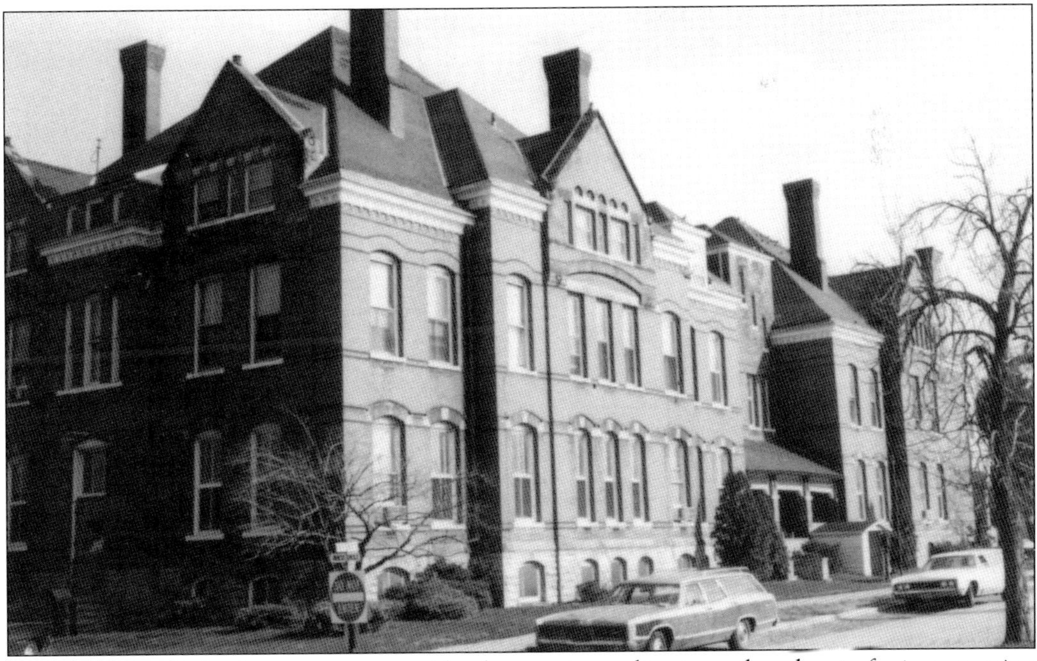

The old hospital's final years were met with advances in medications, the advent of private nursing homes, and a national shift from institutional care to community-based services. Also, a state auditor's inspection forced the hospital to face its physical condition—dilapidated, decayed, and dangerous buildings and infrastructure, and fire hazards—problems that could not realistically be remedied. It was the beginning of the end for the old state hospital. (NOPH.)

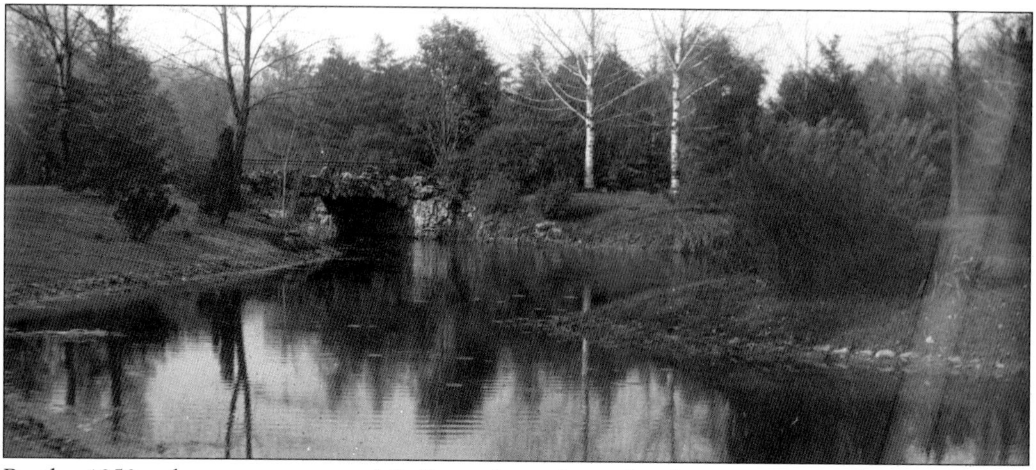

By the 1950s, there was a general feeling of new hope for the recovery of the mentally ill. While treatment methods remained much the same—such as electric shock, insulin coma, and hydrotherapy—knowledge of how to more effectively use them had improved. The key to recovery, however, remained early treatment, and an increase in the number of voluntary admissions helped make treatments more effective as well. (TLCPL.)

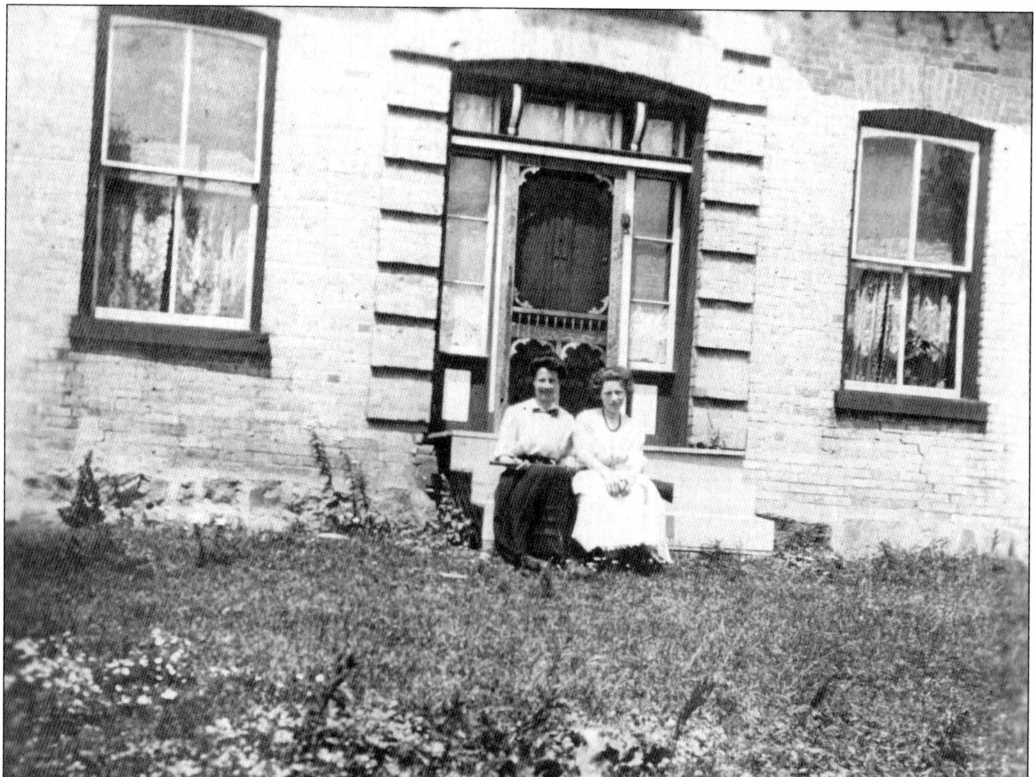

Over the previous decade, the recovery rate for involutional melancholia, or mid-life depression, ballooned to around 90 percent. However, the number of cases of senile dementia also increased as people lived longer and the general population aged. Dr. Duty explained that this would continue to be a problem until more was learned about "hardening of the arteries." (TLCPL.)

The number of paresis cases had declined as the new antibiotic penicillin became available and was used to treat syphilis. Paresis is a partial or general paralysis that occurs in the later stages of the disease when it attacks the brain and nervous system. Success in the early treatment of syphilis with penicillin allowed the hospital to discontinue the use of malarial fever therapy. (TLCPL.)

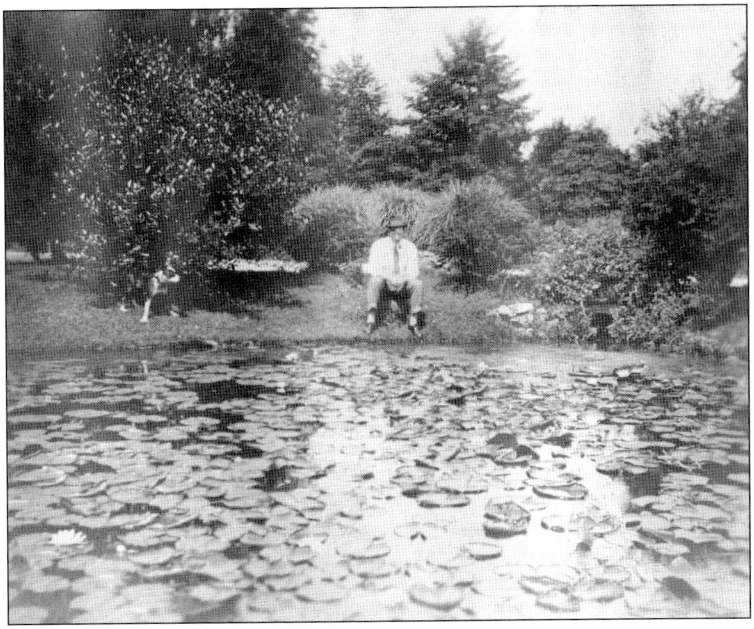

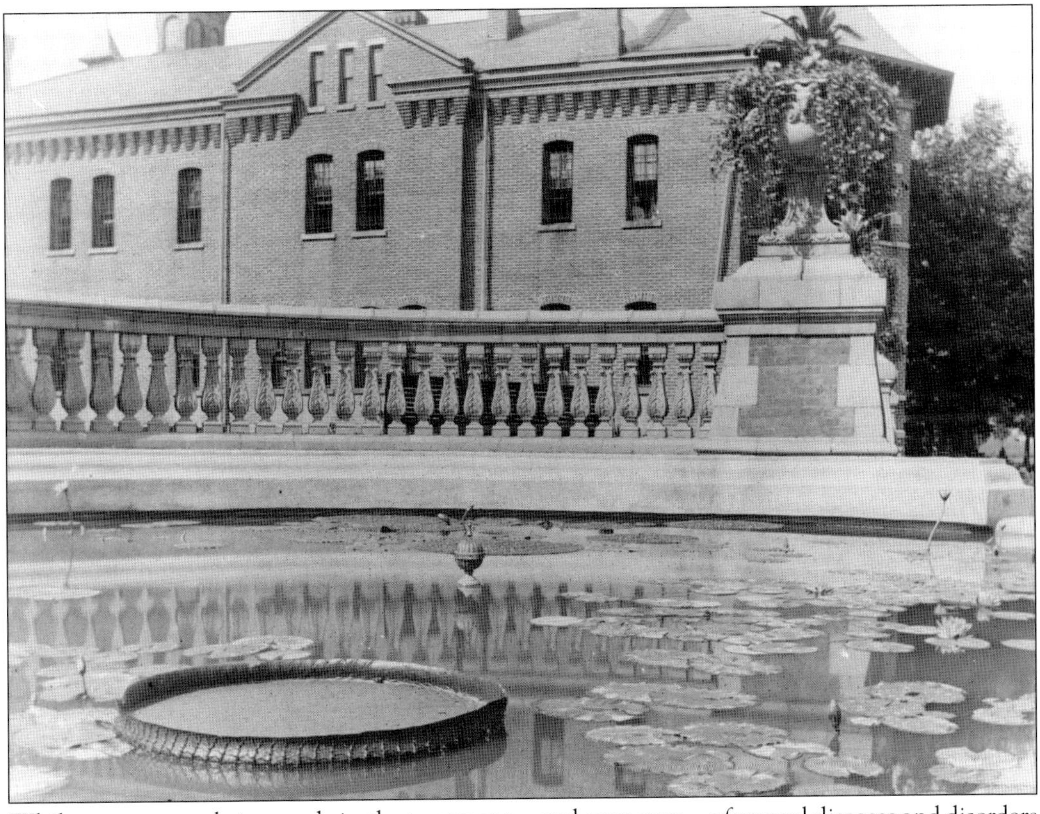

While progress was being made in the treatment—and even cure—of several diseases and disorders at this time, others emerged and became more prevalent than before. Schizophrenia, while present before, now became a major issue at the hospital, and cases of manic-depressive psychoses and hypochondria were also on the rise. (TLCPL.)

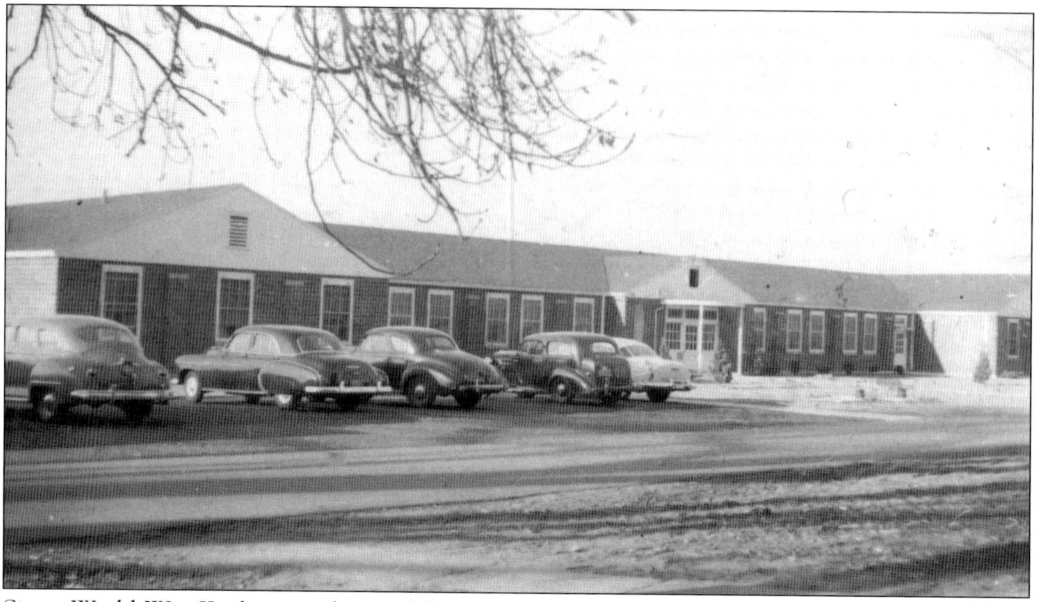

Since World War II, the state hospital had become a dumping ground for the aged who could no longer be cared for at home. As a response to this new and overwhelming issue, the hospital opened Cottage 14 specifically for geriatric patients in 1953. Later nicknamed the "death house," it was remembered by all who worked or visited there for its horrible odor. (TLCPL.)

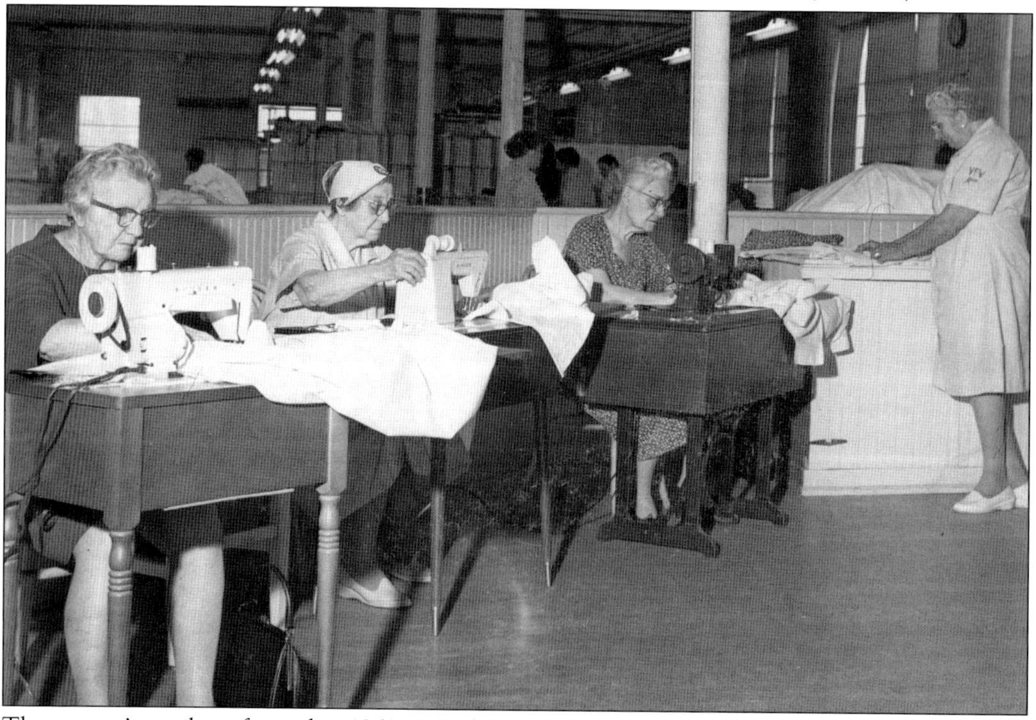

The women's auxiliary formed in 1950, one of only a few charitable groups in the country affiliated with mental institutions. Soon after its formation, the group organized chapters in Fulton and Ottawa Counties and had plans to do the same in all of the counties in northwest Ohio served by the hospital. (NOPH.)

The women's auxiliary's mission was to support the doctors' and nurses' work and assist them with tasks, stamp out stigma by holding programs to educate the public about mental illness, and raise money to provide improvements needed at the hospital and supply items for patient comfort not included in the hospital's budget. (NOPH.)

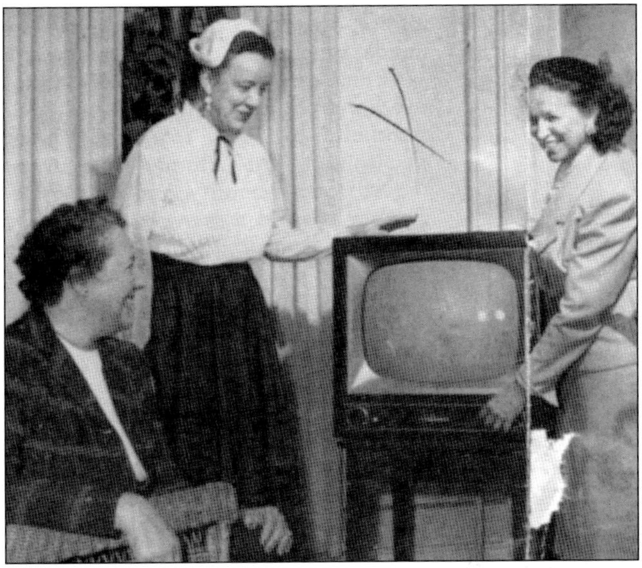

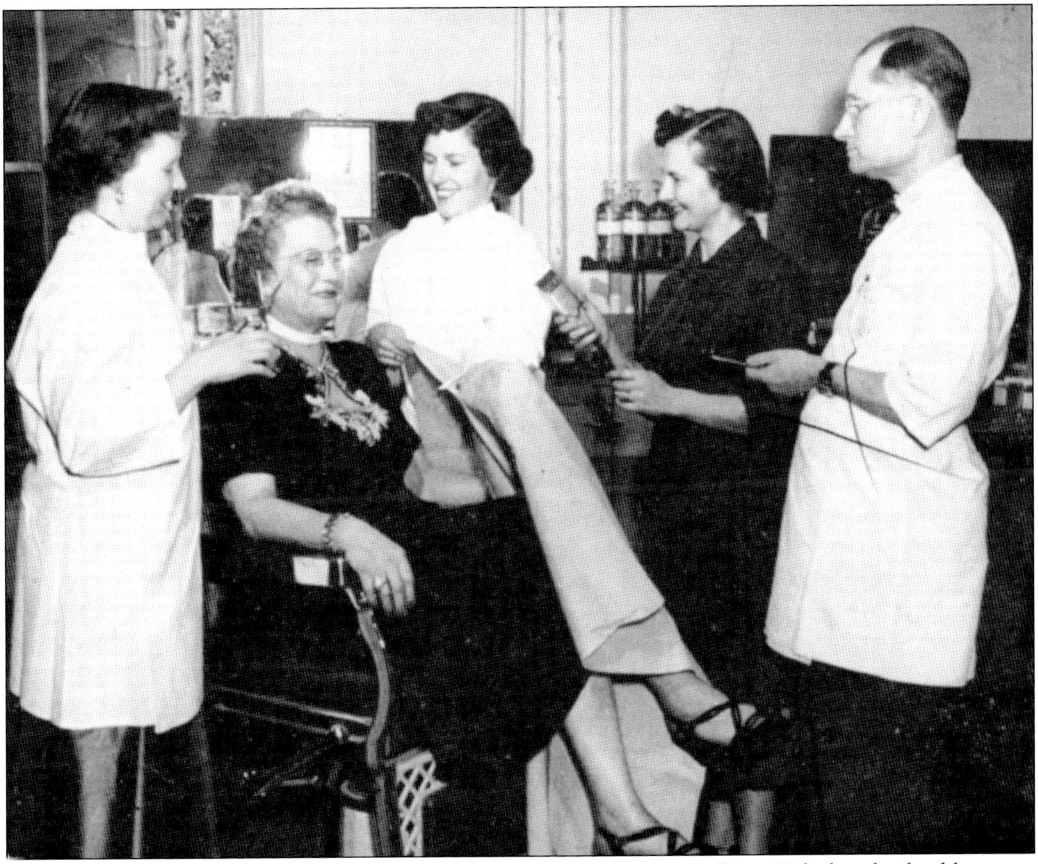

One of its first fundraisers was a show by Theresa Breuer, a singer from Toledo who had become famous for her TV, stage, and radio shows. Other events included a series of monthly square dances at the hospital and a Patron's Dance. With the proceeds from these events, the group installed a barbershop in Cottage 10 in 1951. (NOPH.)

T-rimming S-urely H-elps

Thanks to all the fair ladies
of Auxiliary fame!!
We now have a Barber Shop
In fact as well as name.

If you harbor any doubts,
Just do as we have done—
Watch BOB CASHEN do his work,
You'll find it lots of fun.

With clippers or with scissors
(It matters not to him)
When he gets thru you will find,
You've really had a trim.

That boy can surely "clip" them,
Not as the gangsters do,
But as you would like it done—
It'll thrill you thru and thru.

Just a clippity clip, clip,
And a fast snip or two.
The job is done P.D.Q.
And at NO COST to you.

****

Now for our WONDERFUL Shop—
It is a work of ART;
And mighty well it should be
For it sprang from the HEART.

***********Anonymous.

The barbershop was well received and much appreciated by patients and staff. This poem was written about the barbershop by an anonymous person, probably a patient. The project had such a positive effect that the auxiliary began working to raise money for a beauty shop for female patients. (NOPH.)

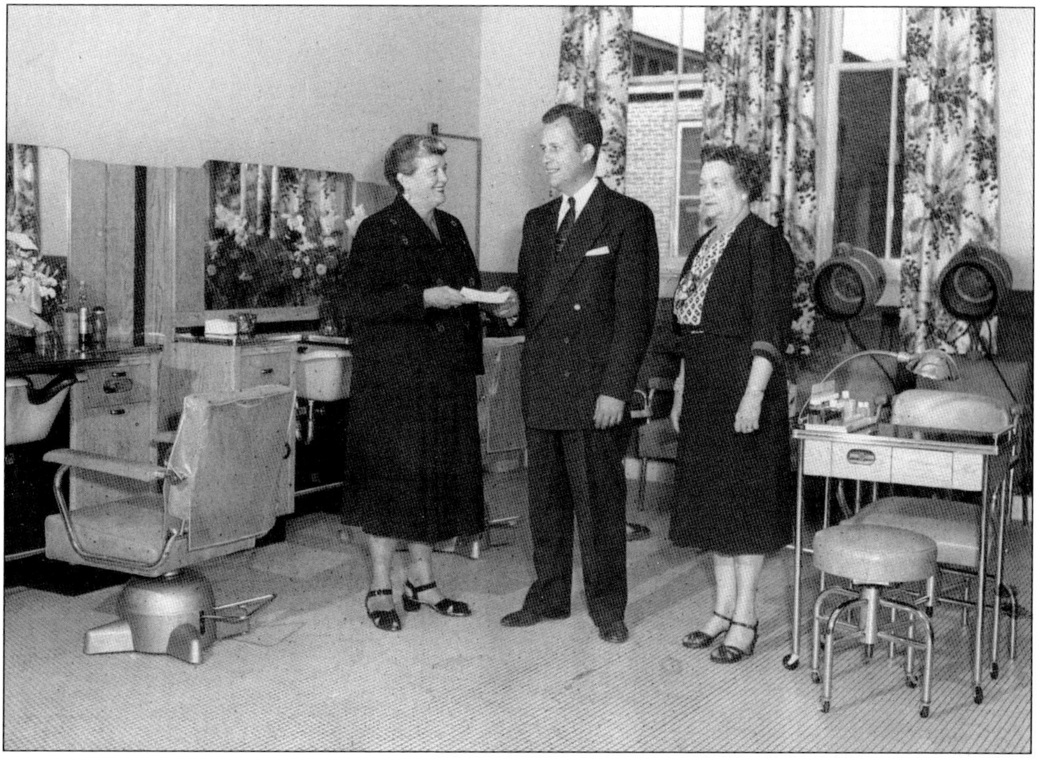

The beauty salon was paid for by the auxiliary, and installed and dedicated in the Receiving Hospital in 1953. The salon was equipped to provide the same level of services available in commercial shops in the community. Since interest in caring for one's personal appearance is an indicator of healthy thinking, it was also therapeutic for the patients. (TLCPL.)

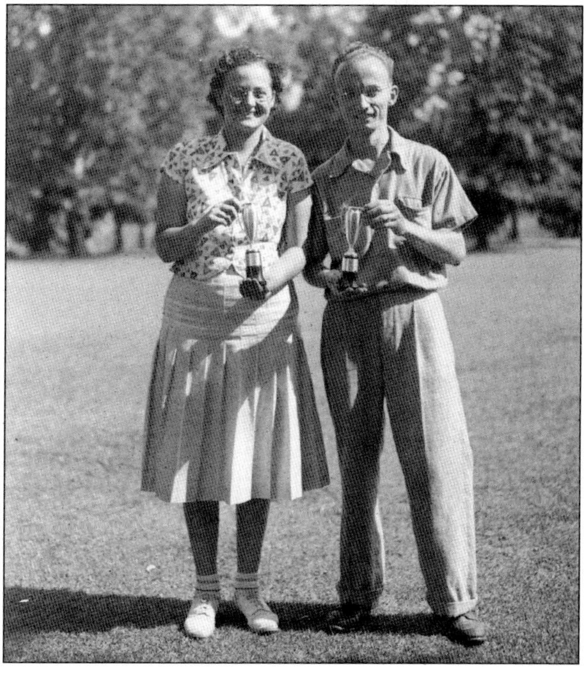

Originally, the nine-hole golf course was for use by patients and staff only. In later years, however, the women's auxiliary held a public tournament there to raise money for the hospital's benefit. In 1951, a two-day event, open to both men and women, was held to honor Toledo amateur and golf course architect Harold Weber. Pictured here on the course are Fred Bigelow Jr. and an unidentified woman. (NOPH.)

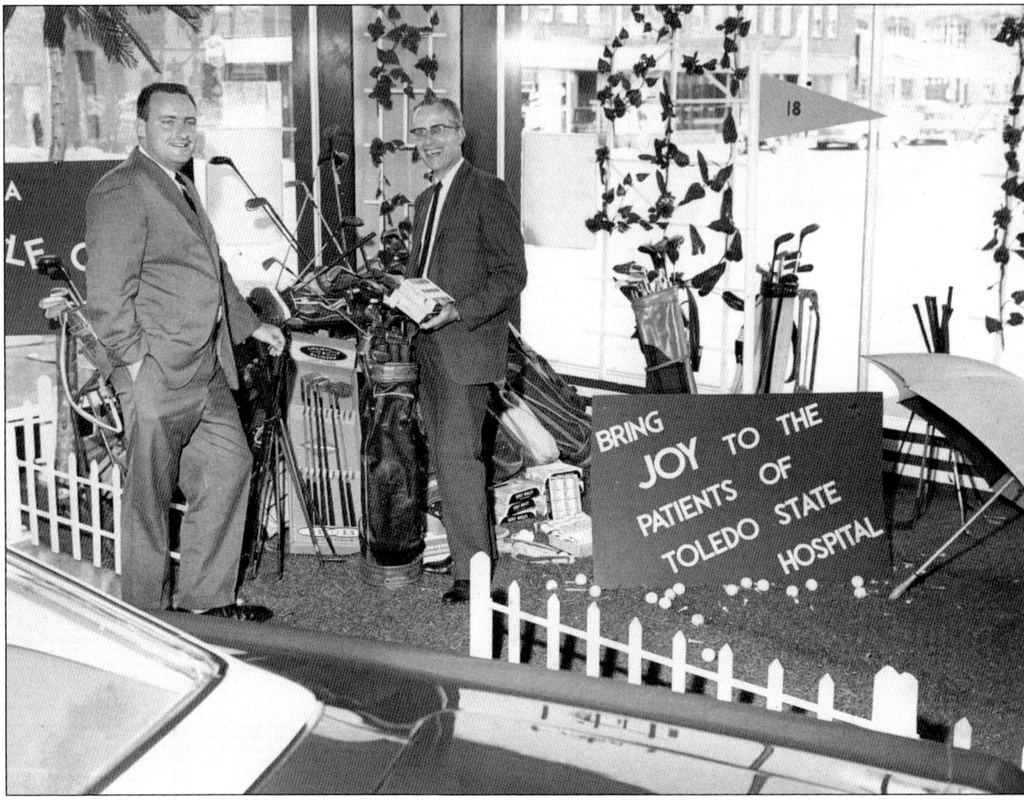
BRING
JOY TO THE
PATIENTS OF
TOLEDO STATE
HOSPITAL
18

In 1966, Toledo golfers donated nearly 50 sets of golf clubs, bags, and balls to the hospital after letters were posted at area courses and sent to club members informing them of the patients' lack of equipment. A local automobile dealership, Jim White Chevrolet, organized and initiated the drive and presented the equipment to Dr. Duty. (NOPH.)

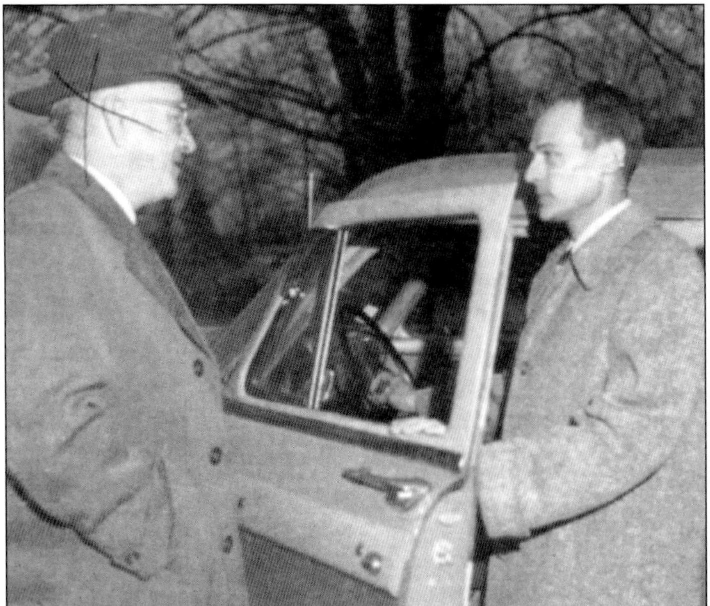

The women of the auxiliary soon recruited their husbands and male friends and organized a men's auxiliary group. By 1953, membership in both groups totaled 1,200. The men often drove male patients to town for sporting events and provided valuable companionship. The outings helped dispel public prejudice toward hospital patients. The men also helped with the women's fundraising and benefit projects. (NOPH.)

During the holiday season, the auxiliary sold Christmas trees and wreaths, and other holiday-related crafts made by its members. The money raised from these sales was used to pay for the annual patient Christmas party. Each year, they also collected, purchased, and wrapped a Christmas gift for every patient at the hospital. In 1965, the group distributed 2,700 gifts to patients. (NOPH.)

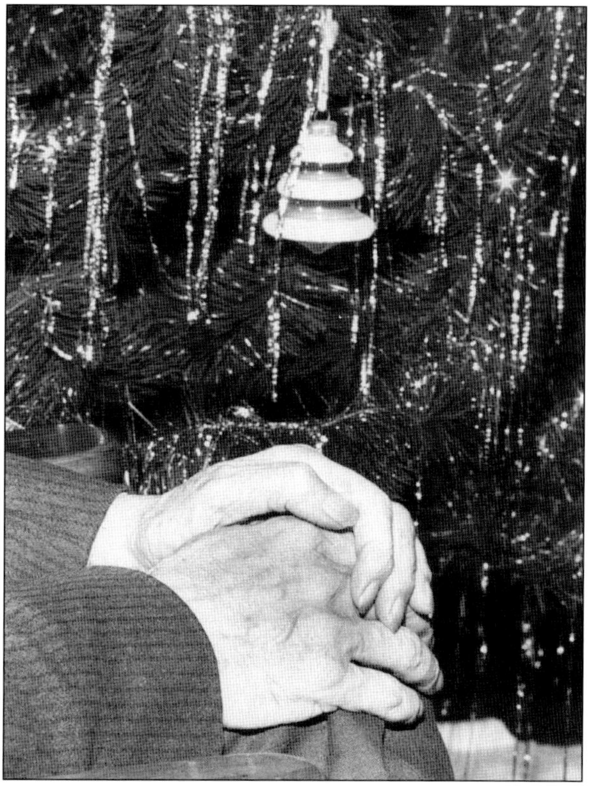

The first wing of the new Receiving Hospital was completed in 1948, and the two west wings in 1952. The last wing, built in 1958, brought the hospital's capacity to 220. It was intended to serve the approximately one million people in northwest Ohio, and treatments were to be more intense but of shorter duration, thereby reducing costs. (NOPH.)

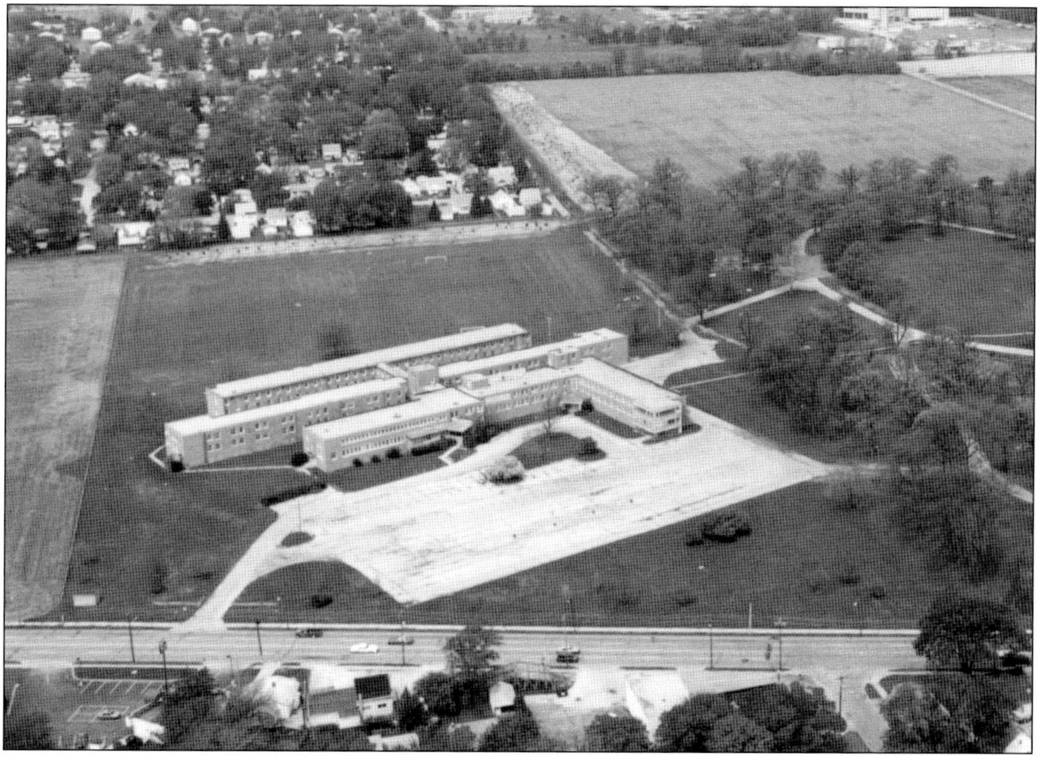

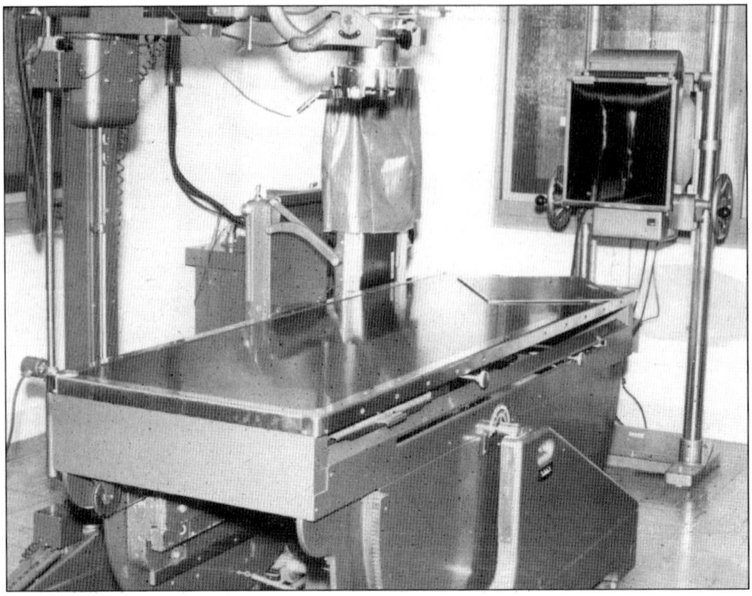

The Receiving Hospital was designed to promote voluntary commitment and emphasize early diagnosis and treatment, when the patient had the best chance of recovering. It was designed to handle short-term cases, and it offered acute medical care services like those available in other hospitals, including an isolation room for those with contagious diseases. (NOPH.)

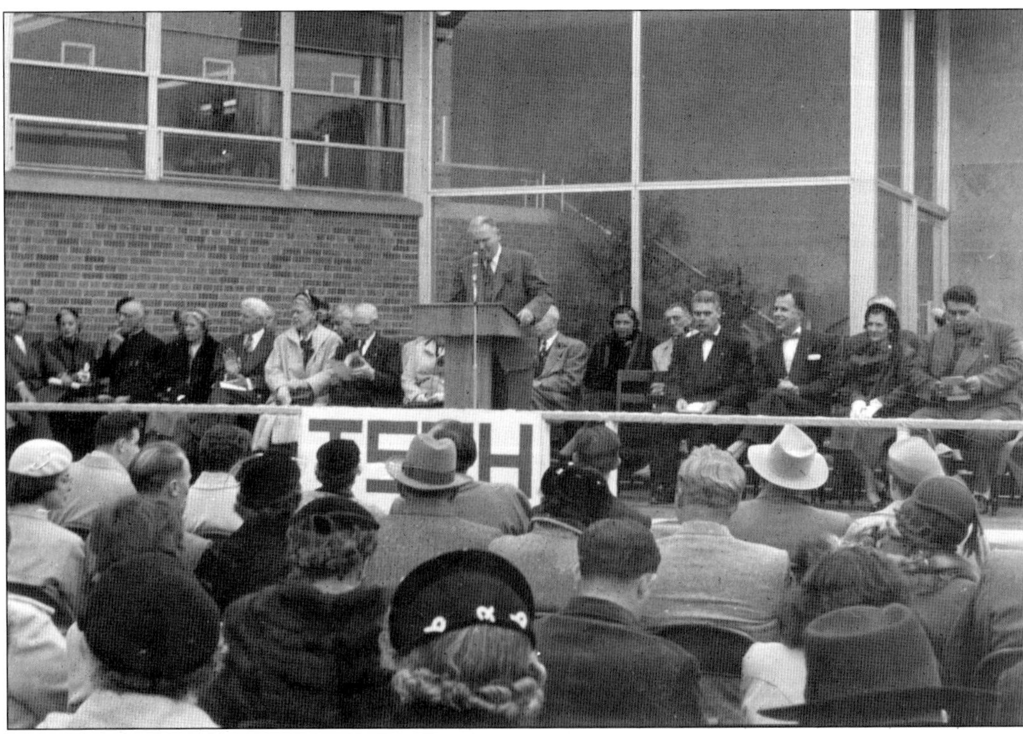

The new hospital was dedicated in a ceremony held November 1, 1952. Judge J.H. Lamneck, state director of public health, gave the dedication speech. This photograph shows Judge Edgar Norris at the podium and Dr. Duty seated third from right. Five hundred people attended the ceremony, and tours of the new building were given afterward. (NOPH.)

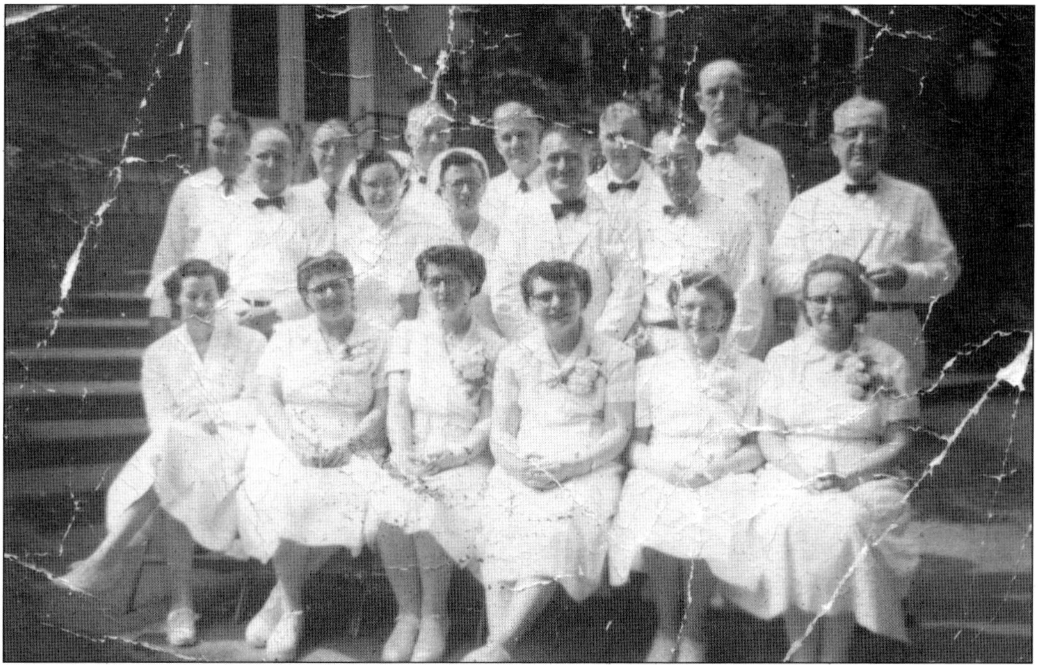

However, while construction of the hospital had been fully funded, no money had been allocated by the state to staff it. It sat unused until October 1953, when a special allocation provided enough money to hire 97 employees to operate the new facility, but only as an extension of the old state hospital, not as a true receiving hospital. (NOPH.)

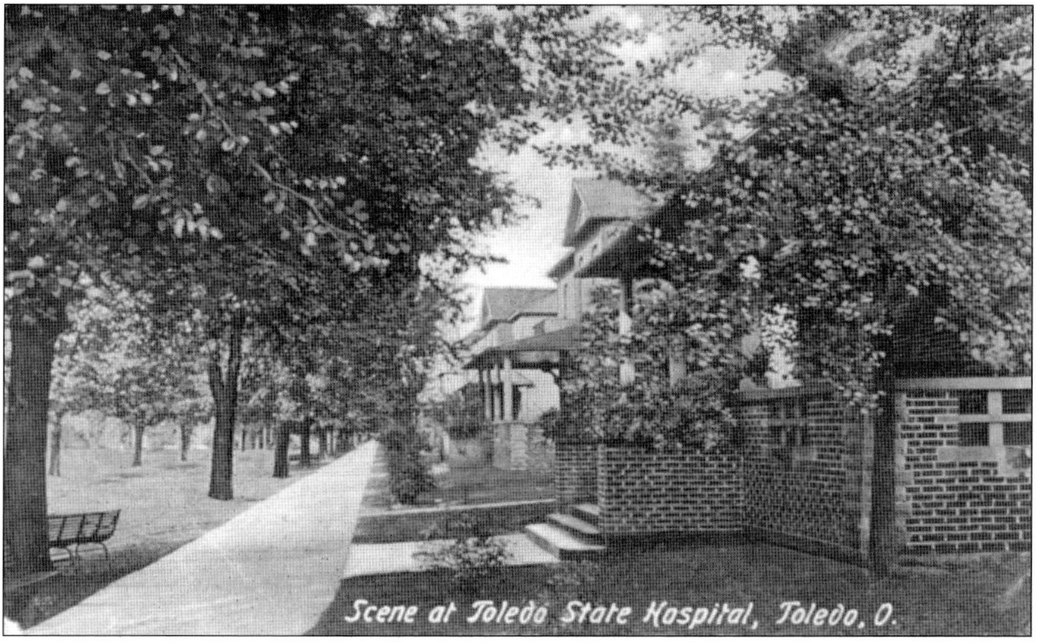

Even after funding for staffing was allocated, it was still not possible to operate the new facility as a receiving hospital. Therefore, people with symptoms of mental illness who came for the services and treatment methods of a receiving hospital often found themselves confined in one of the wards or cottages at the old hospital with chronically mentally ill patients. (NOPH.)

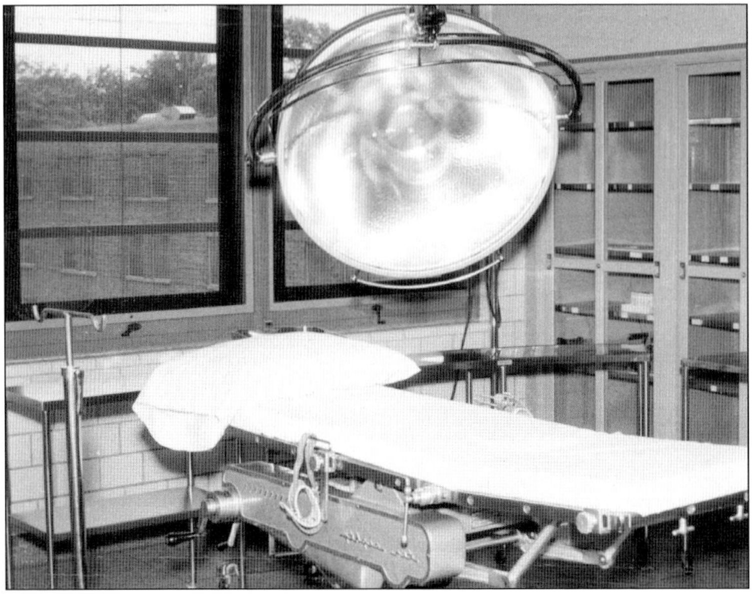

New, state-of-the-art equipment had been installed in the new hospital but also went unused for lack of professional staff to operate it. It had a fully equipped operating room, an x-ray department, a laboratory, a darkroom, examination rooms, and a doctors' lounge. Its large conference room, however, was used as a classroom for nurses' training and a meeting room for the women's auxiliary. (NOPH.)

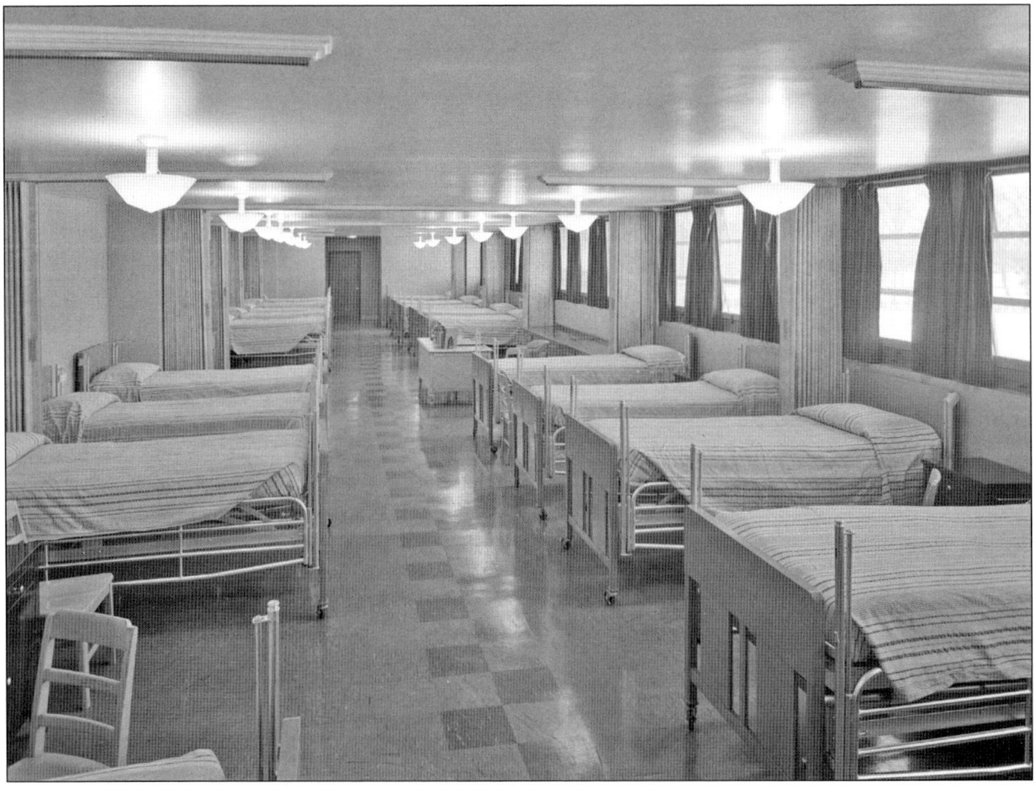

Privacy was a priority in the design of the new Receiving Hospital. Most of the patient rooms were single. However, there were large wards that could be divided into several four-bed rooms, using the accordion-style temporary walls shown here. Paint colors were also thoughtfully chosen—calming blues and greens for excitable patients, and vibrant reds and yellows for those who were depressed. (TLCPL.)

Social interactions were strongly encouraged, especially for the depressed. Kitchenettes and dining rooms were available for patients who wished to prepare light food for small parties of visiting family and friends. Even though the Receiving Hospital was new, it immediately began to show signs of damage from settling and lack of maintenance, as evidenced by the peeling walls in the kitchenette shown here. (NOPH.)

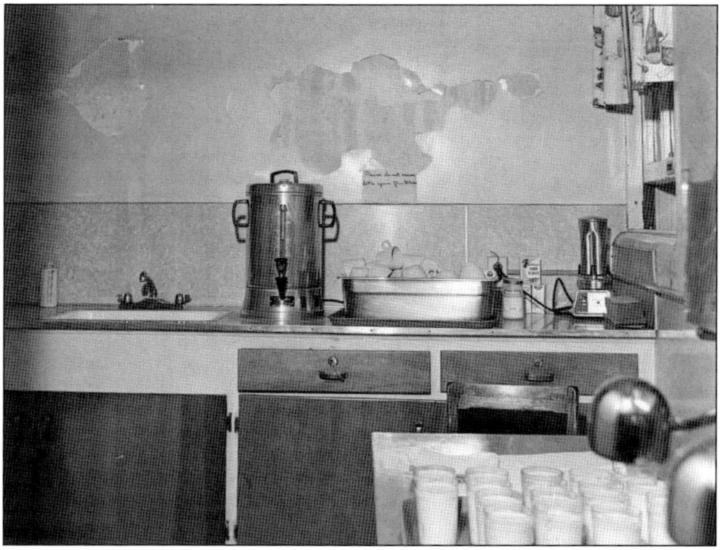

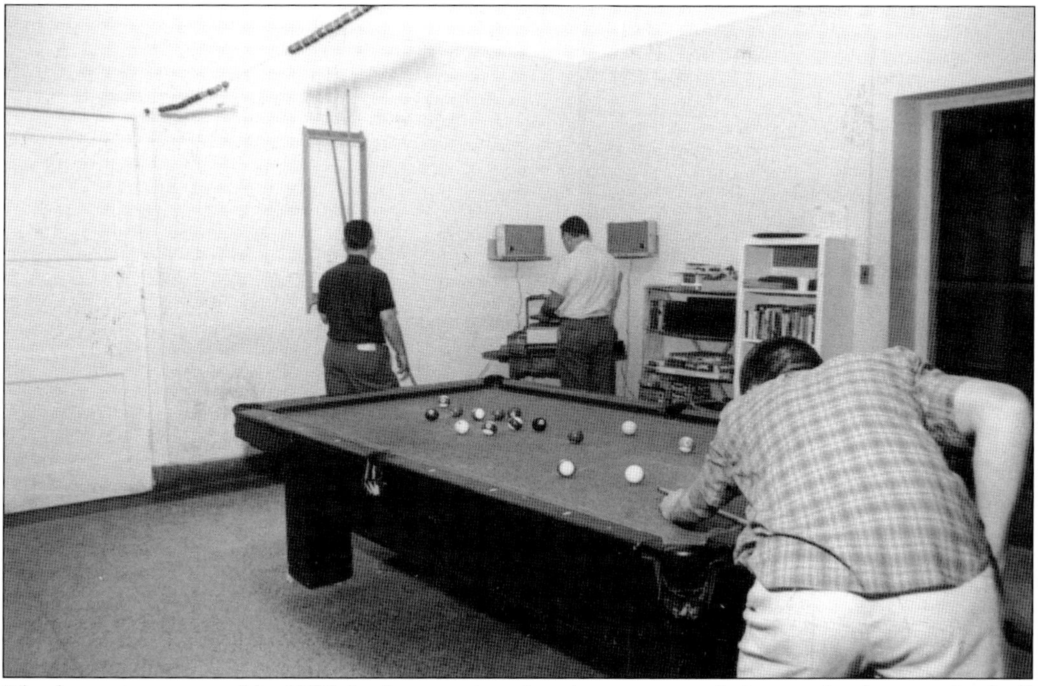

The last wing, opened in 1958, had recreational and occupational therapy facilities, a day hall with a TV and radios, a patient cafeteria, and a music room with a piano and a phonograph. Pictured here is the men's recreation room. The Receiving Hospital would only be used for about 40 years before being phased out and demolished in the 1990s. (TLCPL.)

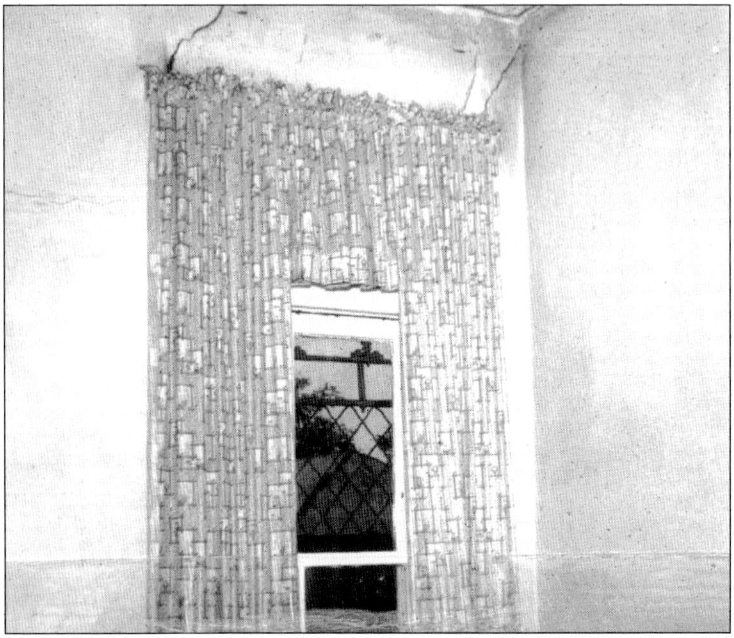

Ohio state auditor James A. Rhodes conducted an inspection of the Toledo State Hospital's facilities from 1954 to 1957. Three major issues were cited consistently: crumbling buildings and infrastructure, fire hazards, and neglect. Built on quicksand, almost every structure had suffered damage from settling, and some were unsafe. Inadequate financial support had resulted in neglect, and their age made it nearly impossible to bring the buildings up to fire safety standards. (NOPH.)

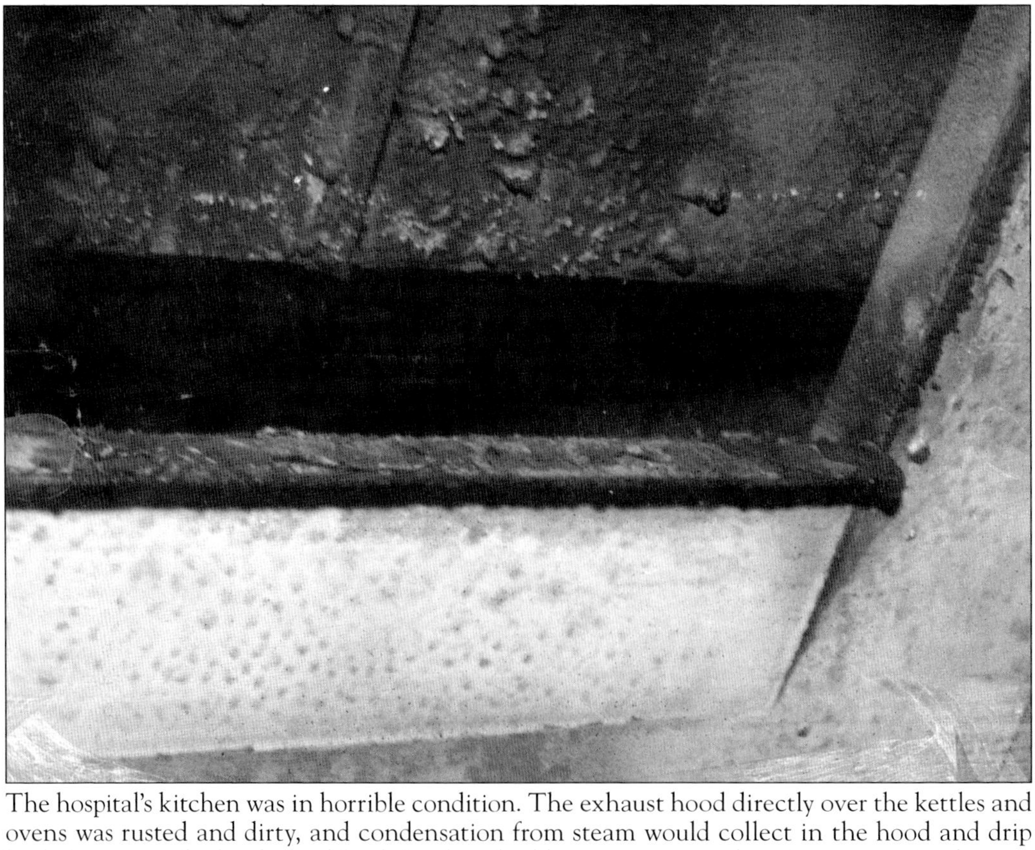

The hospital's kitchen was in horrible condition. The exhaust hood directly over the kettles and ovens was rusted and dirty, and condensation from steam would collect in the hood and drip back down into the kettles and food. Steel worktables were rusty, and equipment was inadequate for the job. (NOPH.)

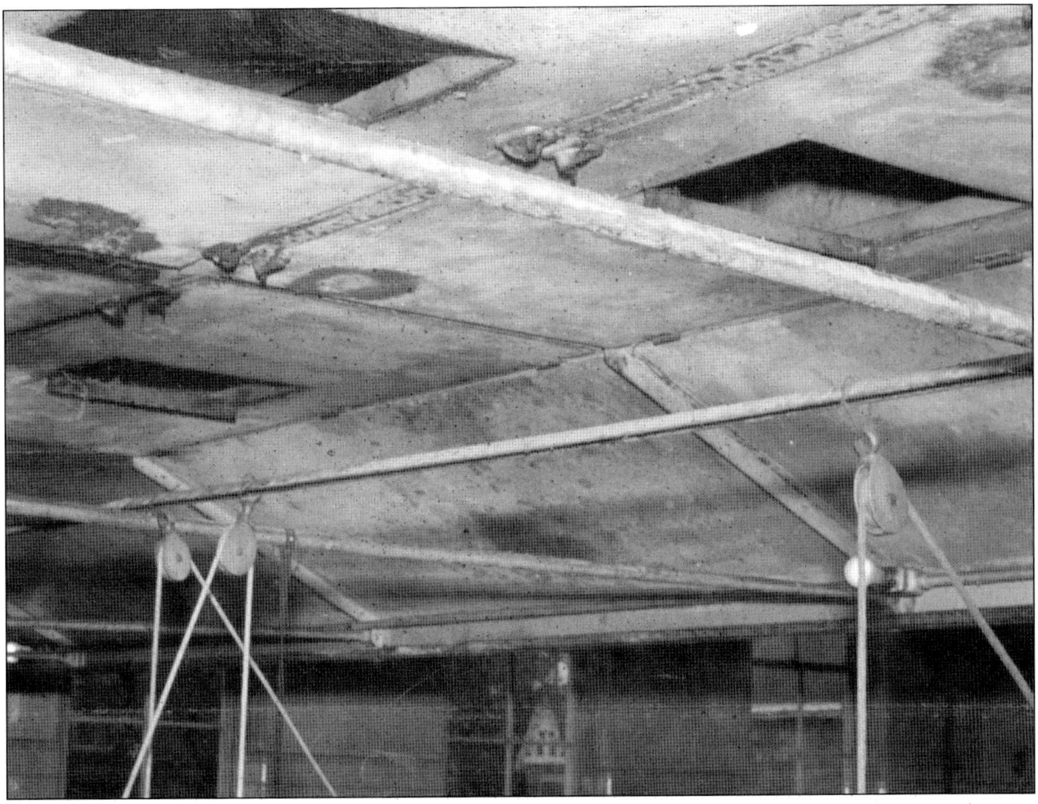

Overhead ductwork was dirty and coated and dripping with grease from years of accumulation. This presented a fire hazard. Plaster was damaged, and the floors were worn out and could not be cleaned. The kettles were worn out and leaked liquid from the food being cooked in them. The old ovens were in poor condition and often upset the food being baked. (NOPH.)

The pots-and-pans washing room was also in poor condition. The sinks were of iron and had rusted through. The floor was dirty, and the clean pans were washed and placed on the floor, leaning against a wall to dry. The vegetable paring room was also in poor condition with worn-out wooden tables to work on. Fifty women worked in this room. (NOPH.)

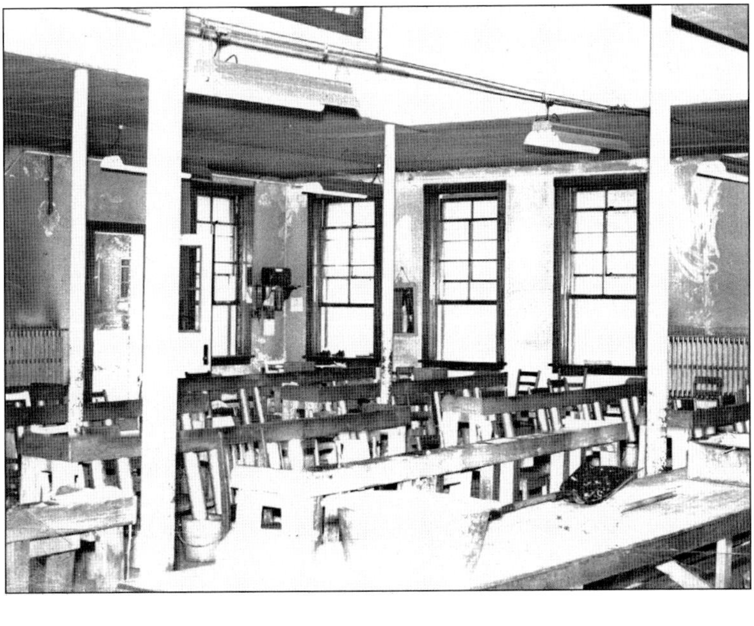

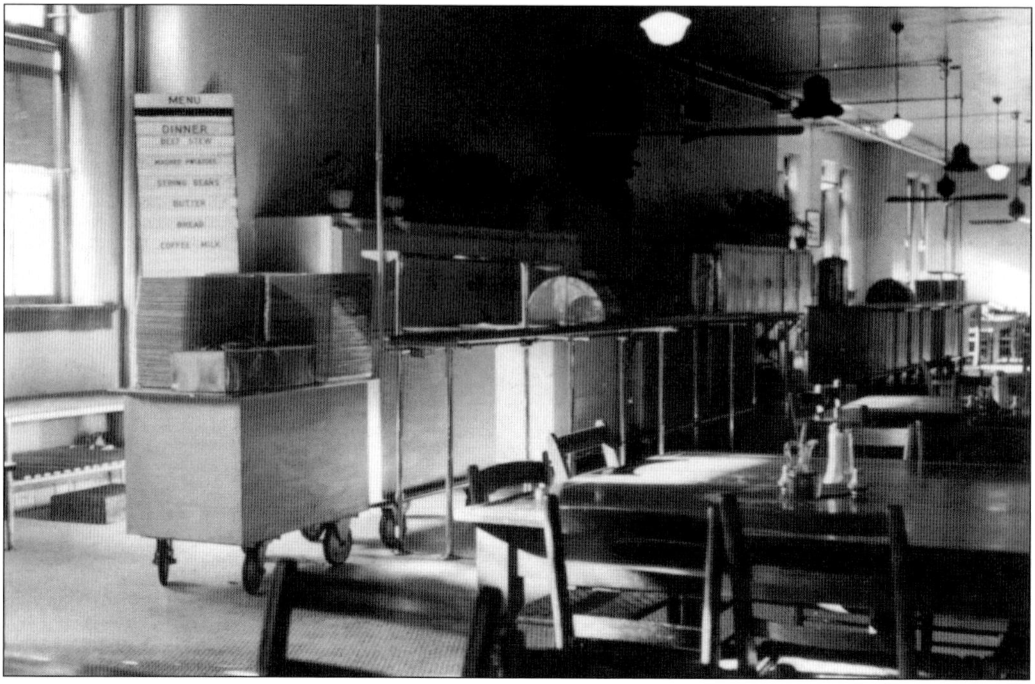

The patient cafeteria was located across the street from the Administration Building. It was in poor condition and needed new floors and ceilings. The walls also needed to be patched and painted. The report stated that it would take a lot of work to make this facility a pleasant place to take meals. This photograph is of a later, improved patient cafeteria. (NOPH.)

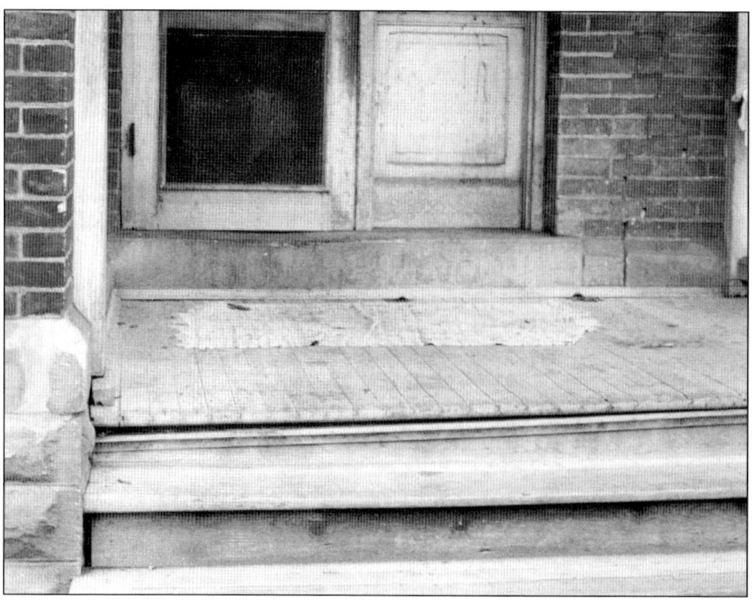

Auditor Rhodes wrote in his report, "On every side at Toledo State Hospital, decay rot and neglect are plainly noticeable." He later stated that "ancient, decrepit buildings and dirty, rusty equipment at Toledo State Hospital make adequate patient treatment impossible," and that "buildings are filthy firetraps, unsanitary, and generally dilapidated." (NOPH.)

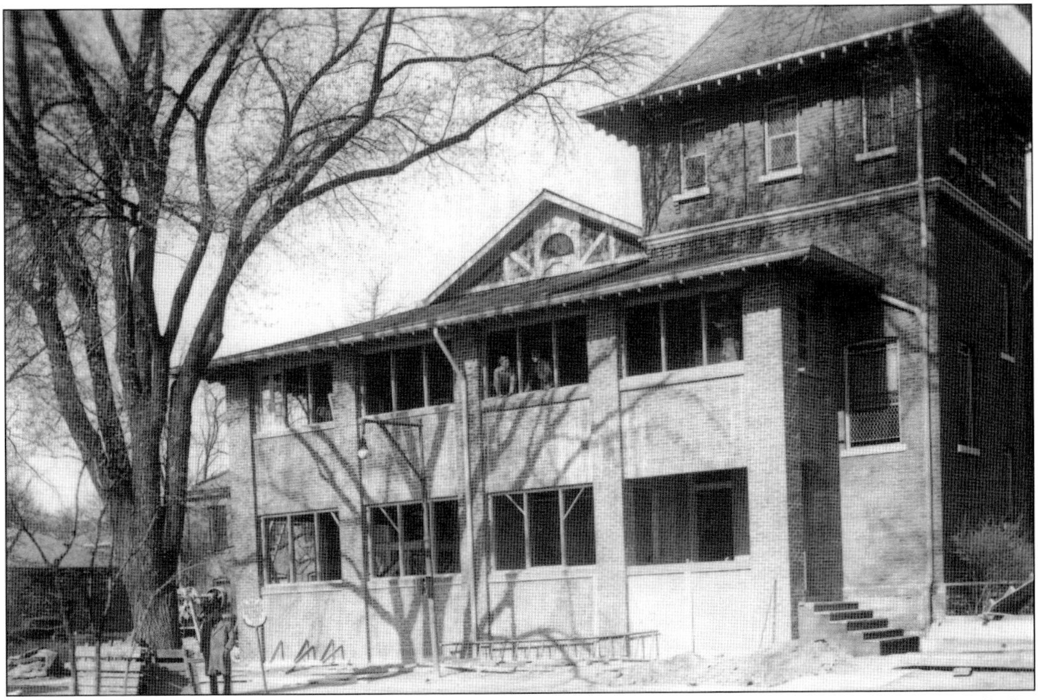

Another major issue related in the auditor's report was inadequate fire safety provisions. Of all the buildings at the hospital, only four had metal fire escapes. None other than the new Receiving Hospital were of fireproof construction, and firehoses had not been inspected with any regularity. (NOPH.)

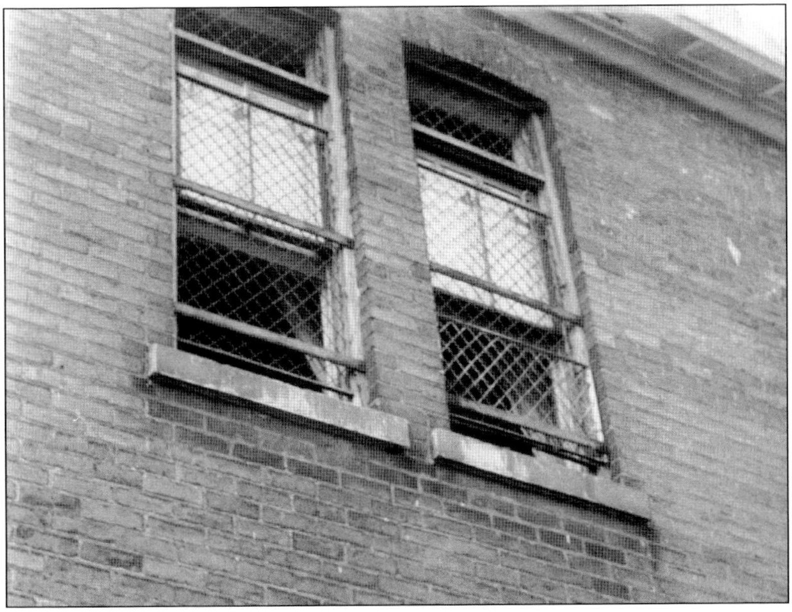

The report pointed out that while most of the cottages had brick exteriors, they were constructed of wood, and over the years, the wood had become very dry. It noted that the dormitories in the cottages were located on the second floor and that the second-story windows were heavily secured with "escape guards." (NOPH.)

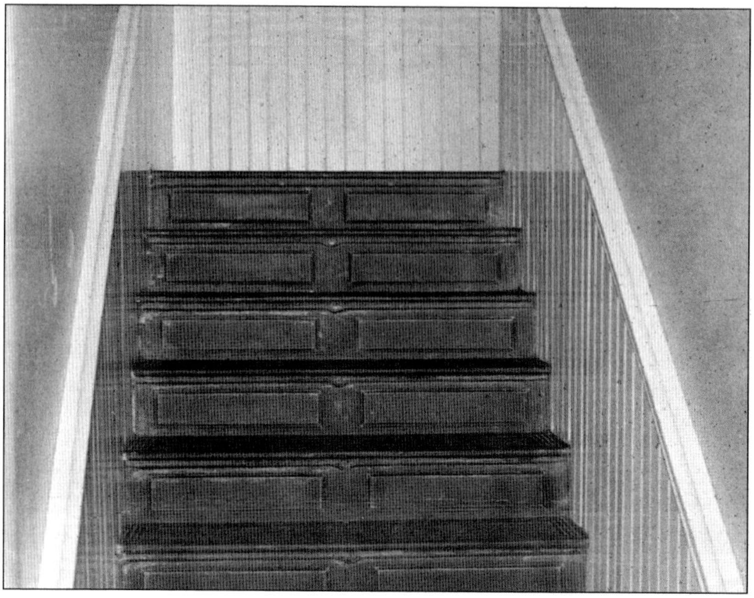

Also of concern regarding the second story dormitories was that each cottage had only one narrow stairway leading from the second to the first floors and that there were no fire escapes. Some of the stairways had metal treads but were constructed of wood. Approximately 55 patients slept in the dormitories in each cottage. (NOPH.)

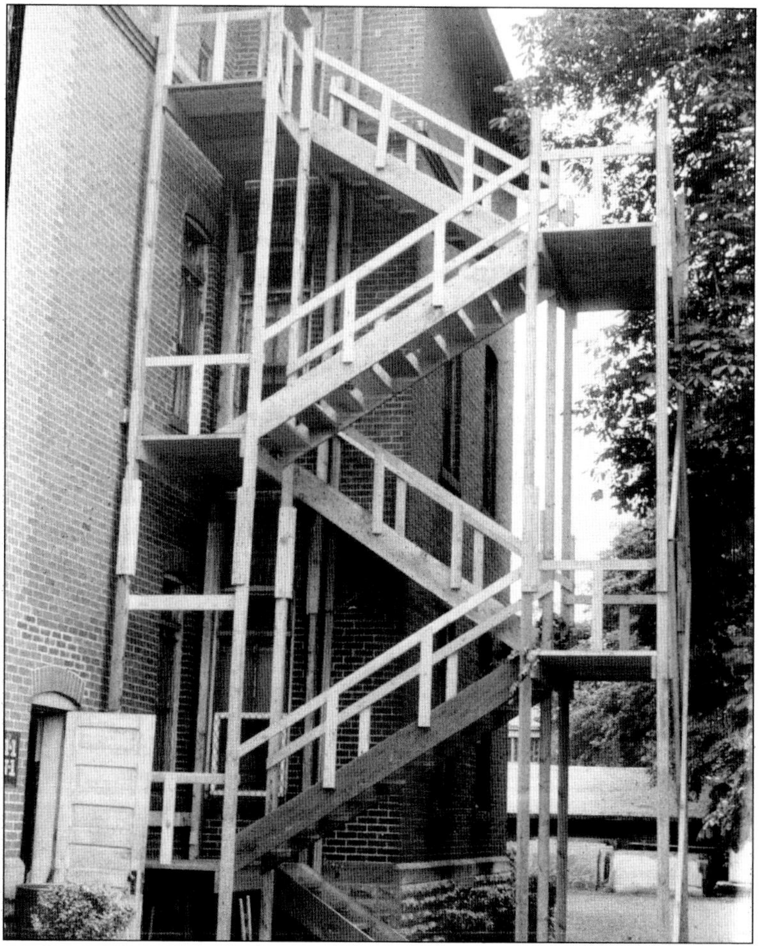

Prior to 1954, the Toledo Fire Department Fire Prevention Bureau conducted an inspection and related many of the same concerns to both hospital administrators and the State of Ohio. The bureau chief asked that metal fire escapes, or wood if metal was not possible, be erected to help firefighters remove patients in case of fire. These wooden stairs were built in 1957. (NOPH.)

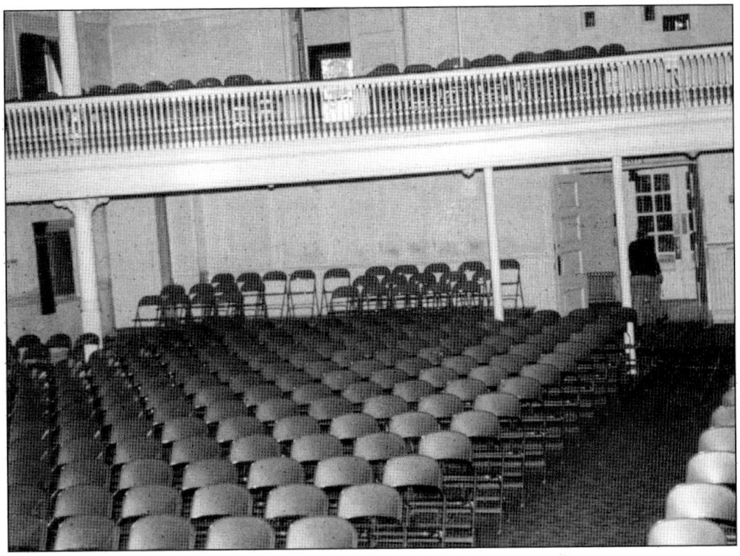

The auditor's inspection found that the walls of the Entertainment Hall had been covered with burlap for acoustical purposes. This was deemed a critical fire hazard. Also, access to extinguishers installed in the building was blocked by stored furniture and equipment. The seating capacity of the hall was 600. It also found cracks around the dome and in the interior walls from settling. (NOPH.)

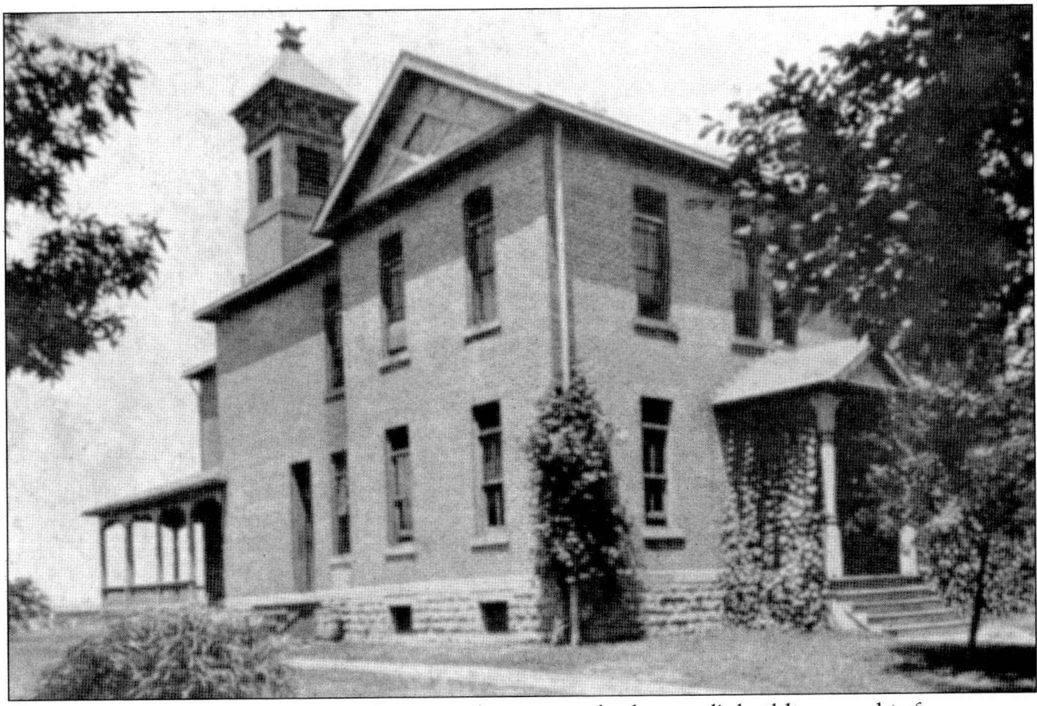

A final area of concern to the auditor was damage to the hospital's buildings and infrastructure from settling. The hospital had been built on land underlaid with quicksand, and cracking walls, foundations, and sagging floors had been a problem almost from the beginning. Cottage 4 had suffered so much damage that it had become unsafe and was abandoned. (NOPH.)

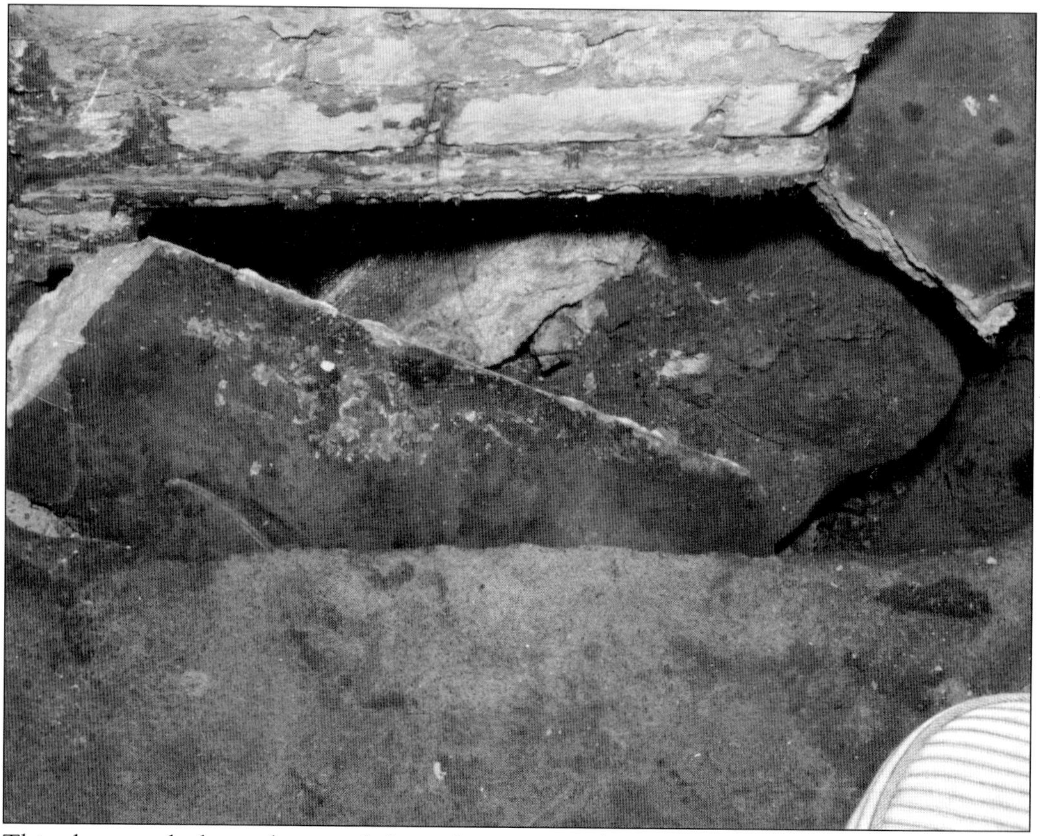

This photograph shows the near failure of a support column in the basement of Cottage 4 due to settling. The hospital's infrastructure suffered as well. A utility tunnel carrying steam pipes to many of the buildings had begun to disintegrate, allowing quicksand to seep in. It had slowly filled to a level that made it very difficult, if not impossible, to work in. (NOPH.)

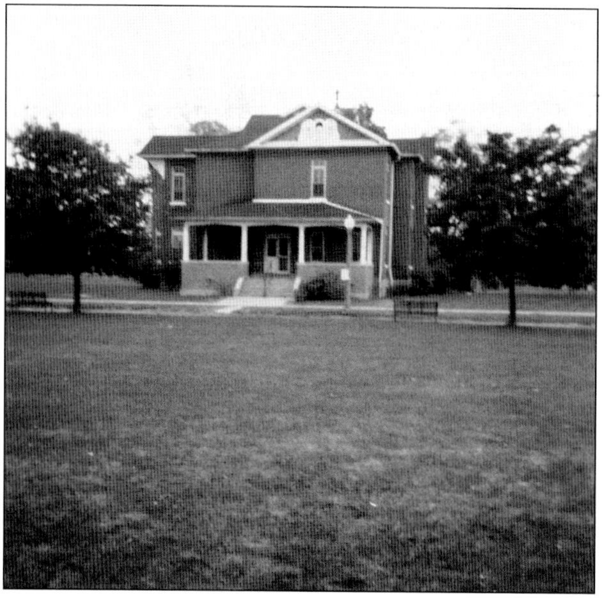

Cottage 3 had also suffered severe damage but was not abandoned. The supports of this building were so weak that the first-floor beams were visibly sagging, and the ceilings were cracking. The second-story floor had taken on the shape of a cone, as it sagged from all four corners. (NOPH.)

The second floor of Cottage 3 was so weak that simply walking across it caused it to shake and the windows to rattle throughout the building. Any bouncing or shaking-type movement caused the beds to vibrate. Fifty-two male patients slept there every night—an estimated four tons of weight on this floor. This photograph is the basement of Cottage 3 and shows the sagging floor overhead. (NOPH.)

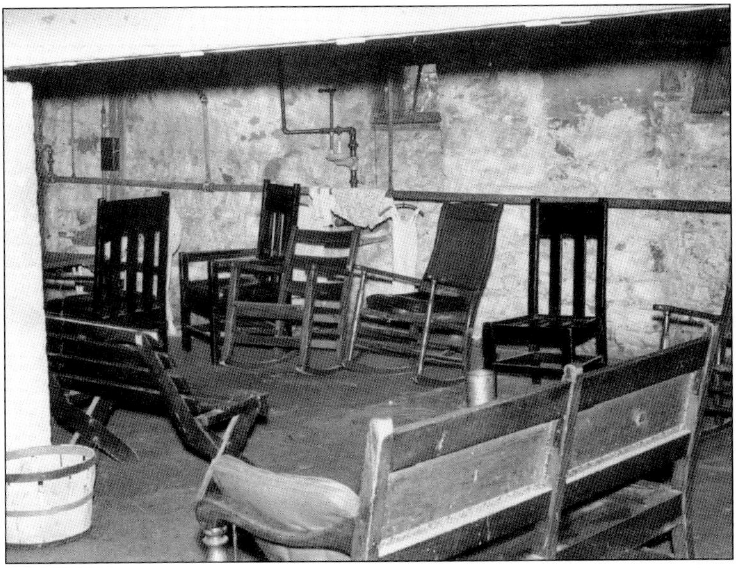

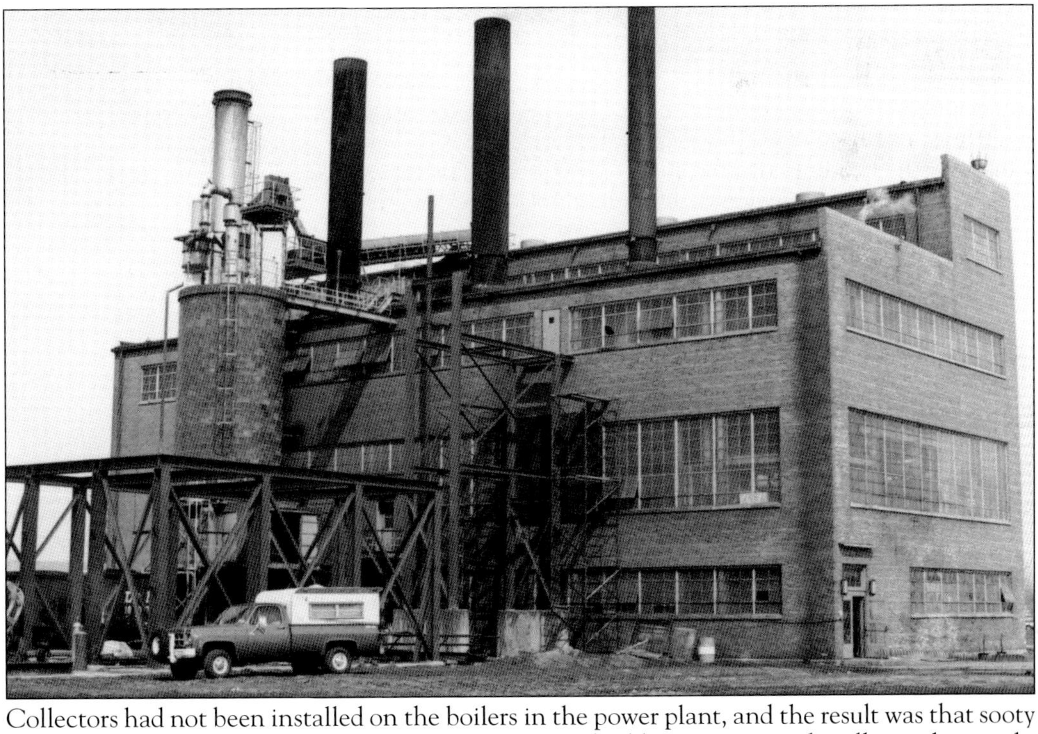

Collectors had not been installed on the boilers in the power plant, and the result was that sooty fallout blackened everything at the hospital, covering buildings, streets, sidewalks, and grounds. Besides presenting a dirty appearance, the fallout clogged gutters, downspouts, and sewers, and caused rust and corrosion to all metal objects that it settled on. (NOPH.)

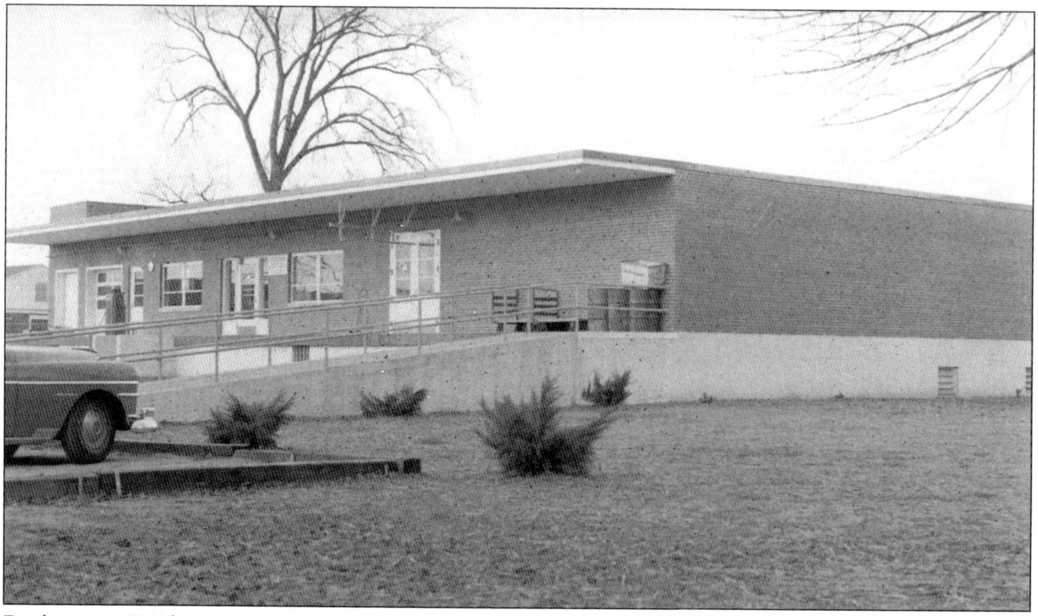

Built in 1955, the Stores Room was reported to be in excellent condition and well managed. The stored supplies and materials were kept well-organized and in clean spaces, and the store manager's records were impeccable. In addition to stores, this building housed the butcher shop and meat coolers. (NOPH.)

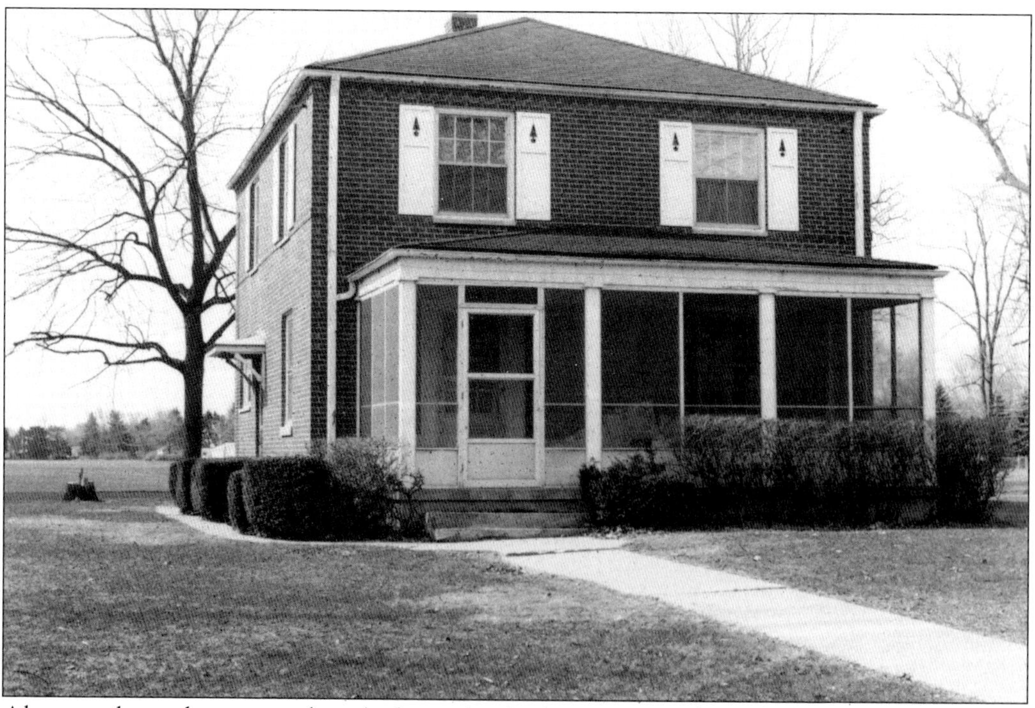

Also noted was that a new three-bedroom brick physician's residence had been built two years earlier but was as of then still unoccupied. Auditor Rhodes cited this as another example of waste, but hospital administration reported that it expected the residence to be filled in July of that year. (NOPH.)

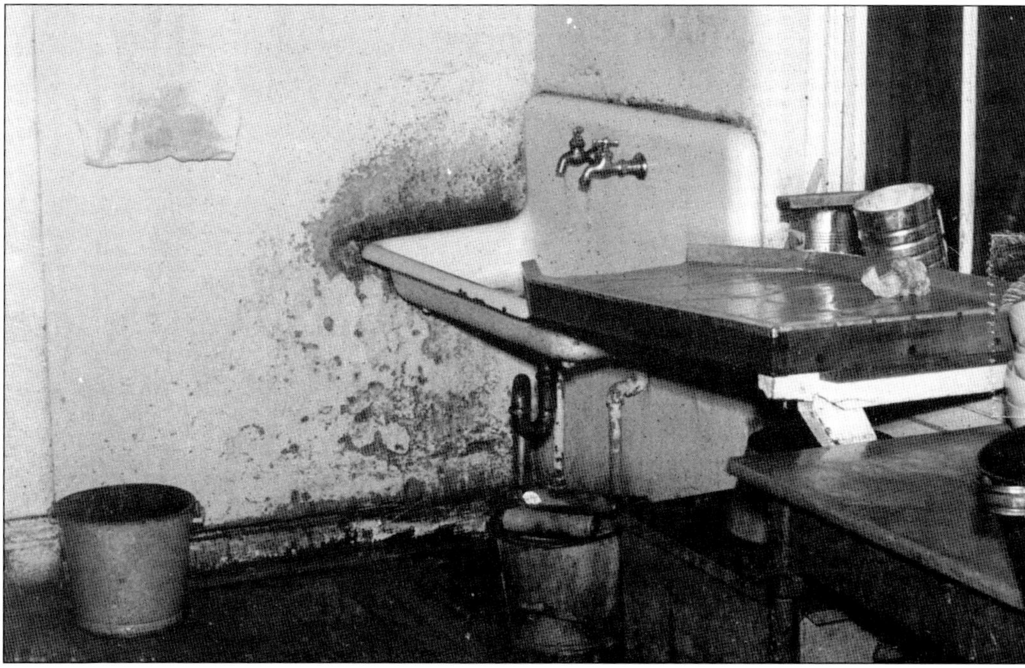

Rhodes did not hold Dr. Duty responsible for the hospital's deplorable condition, but rather blamed the Department of Mental Hygiene and Corrections, as it was responsible for administering the hospital. Dr. Duty, however, blamed the public, saying that lawmakers listen to what their constituents want, but that when it comes to state hospitals, the people in general just do not care. (NOPH.)

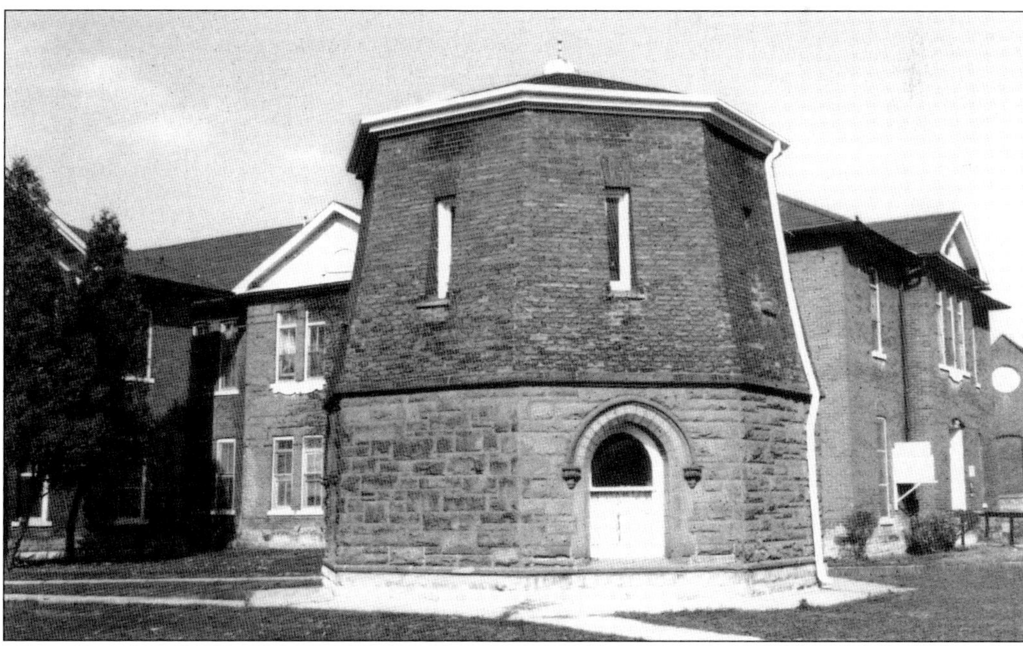

In 1956, the Gothic-style top of the old water tower was removed, and the base was renovated to be used as the hospital's post office. The walls at the base of the tower were said to have been three feet thick. The tower had served as storage for the hospital's water supply for 66 years. (TLCPL.)

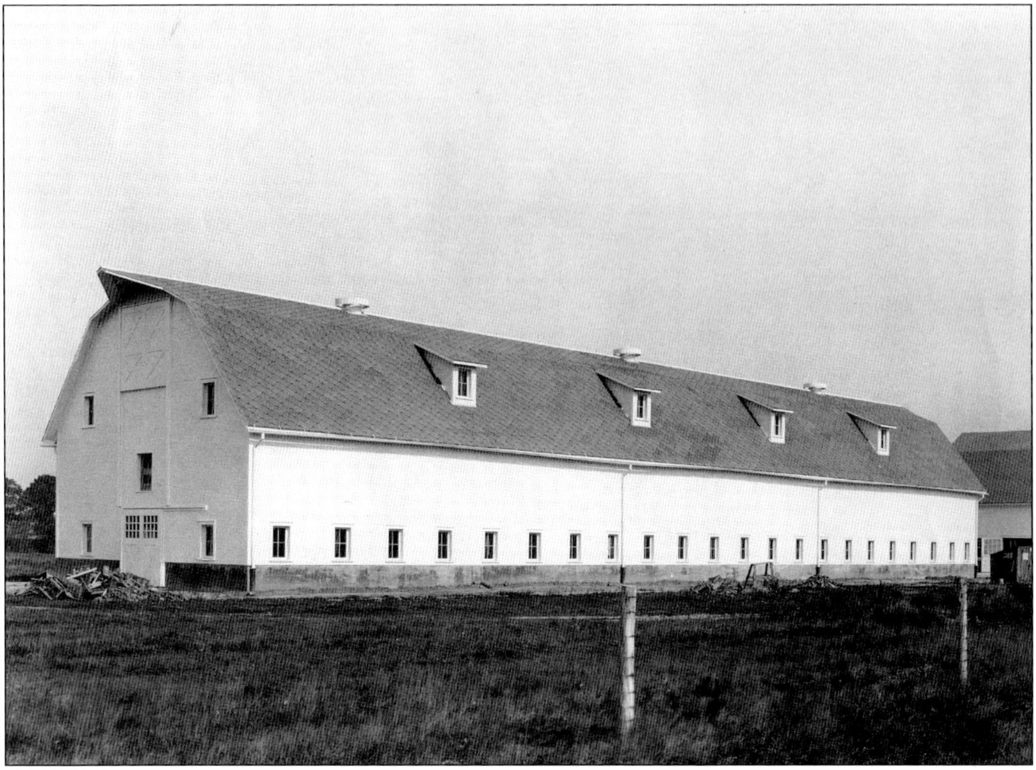

The dairy barn is pictured here around 1957. At this time, the farm had 160 Holstein milking cows, 600 hogs, 1,600 laying hens, and 1,000 pullets. Fifty-five patients worked the farm and cultivated 640 acres. Eight patients tended the piggery. Other farm buildings included heifer, grain, stock, horse, and bull barns and a poultry house. (NOPH.)

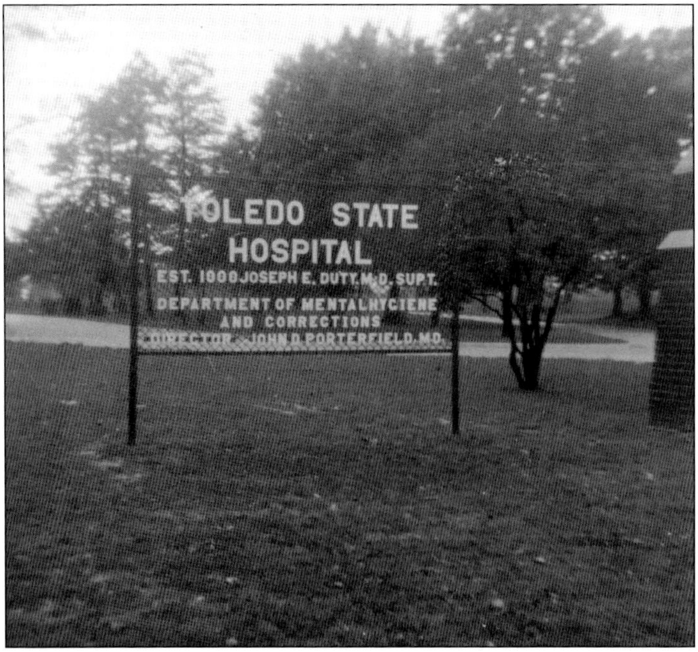
TOLEDO STATE
HOSPITAL
EST. 1888 JOSEPH E. DUTY M.D. SUPT.
DEPARTMENT OF MENTAL HYGIENE
AND CORRECTIONS
DIRECTOR JOHN D. PORTERFIELD M.D.

In October 1957, Dr. Duty was promoted to commissioner of the Ohio Division of Mental Hygiene and moved to Columbus. In November, Dr. Joseph Garland was appointed the new superintendent of the hospital. However, Dr. Duty left his state post in July 1958 due to ill health and, on his doctor's advice, returned to Toledo and to the hospital as superintendent once again. (NOPH.)

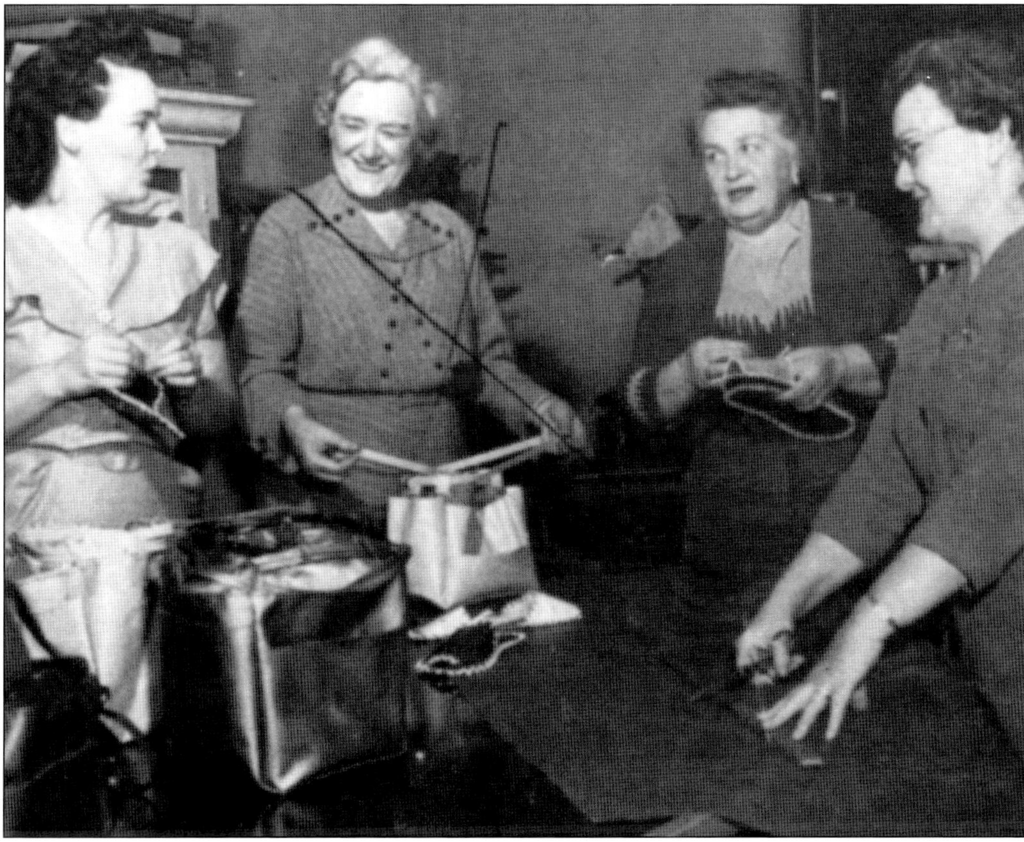

In 1958, the women's auxiliary opened a store in the Occupational Therapy Building. Store fixtures such as clothing racks and shelving were donated by area department stores. Here, the group sold items contributed by members and made by the sewing committee. They also collected gently used children's clothing and ladies' party dresses. (NOPH.)

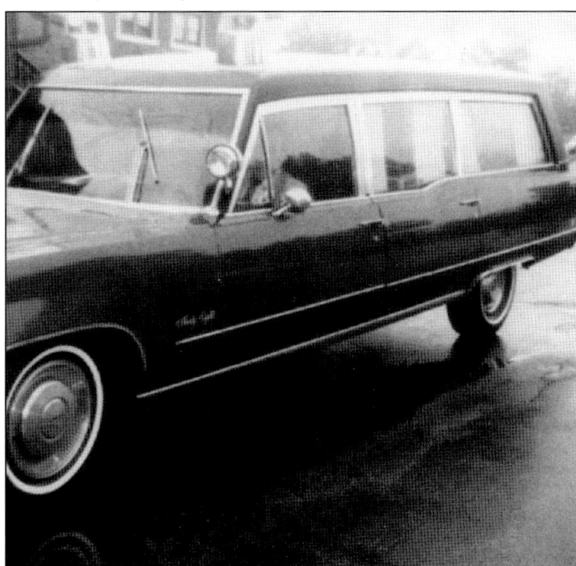

The store was staffed by auxiliary volunteers and was open to patients, staff, and the public one day a week. Proceeds from the store went to purchase equipment needed by the hospital and to repair and replace 60 television sets. The auxiliary was also eventually able to purchase an ambulance for the hospital. (NOPH.)

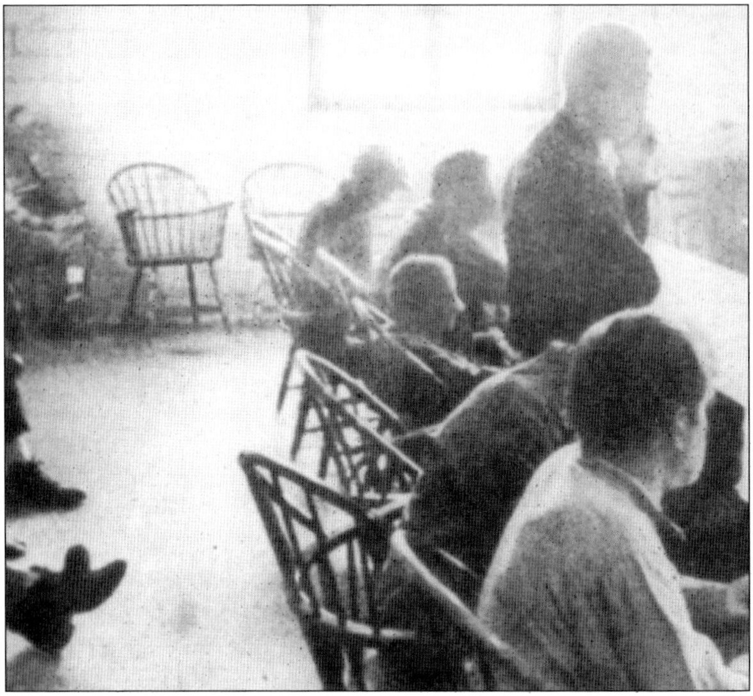

By 1960, the new psychology department was often used for help with the diagnosis and treatment of patients. The psychologists worked directly with the patients, and individual and group therapy were added as treatment options. New medications were the primary means of treatment, and electric shock was still occasionally used. (NOPH.)

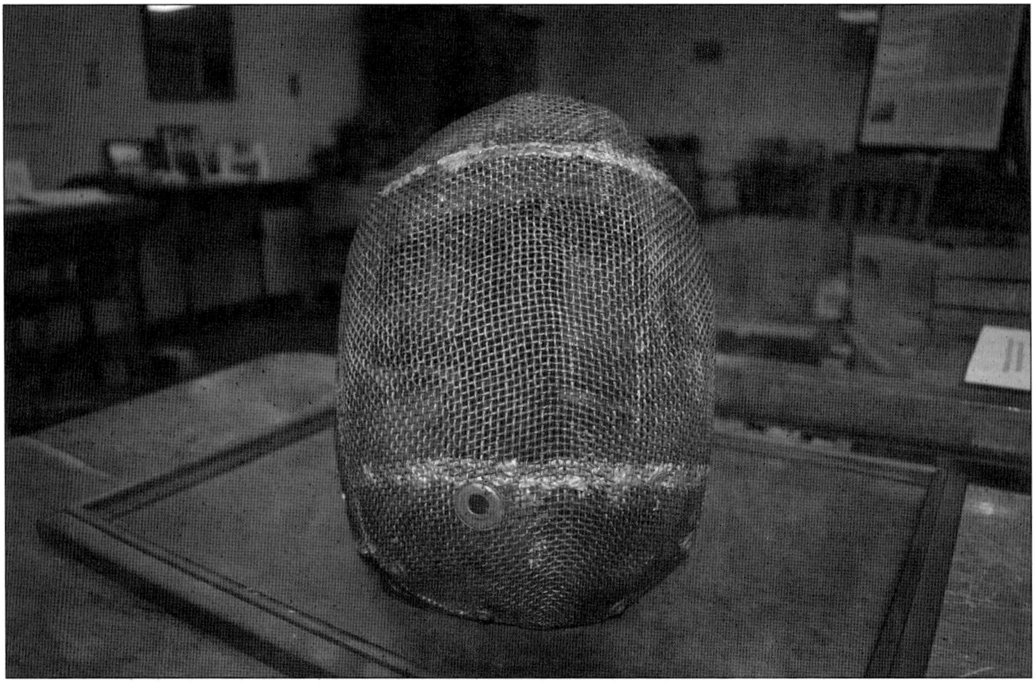

This mask was custom-made for a patient who had an eating disorder known as pica. People with this disorder ingest items that are non-edible, such as dirt, grass, wood, and other such materials that may be harmful. The mask was used on this patient to prevent him from hurting himself—not as a punishment or abuse. (Photograph by author.)

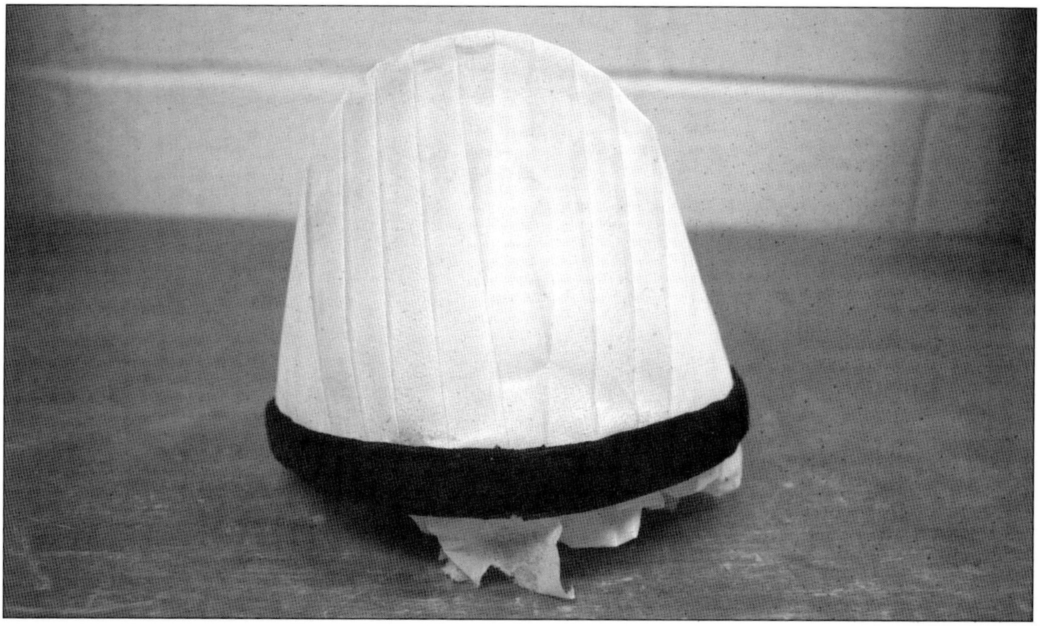

The hospital offered a three-month supplemental psychiatric nursing program to students studying in other hospitals' nursing schools. Some who completed the program were then hired by the hospital. It also began taking medical student residents and psychology and social services interns. This greatly helped alleviate the staff shortage. (Photograph by author.)

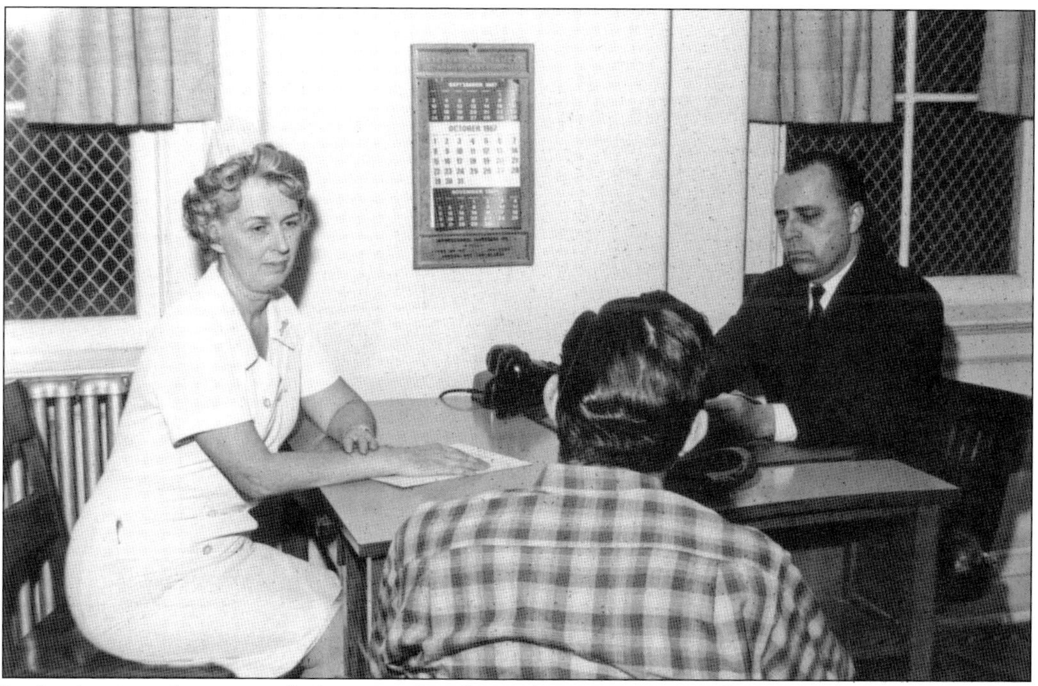

It also instituted a series of educational and enrichment programs for its employees, particularly its attendants, believing that a better-trained staff would improve patient recovery. Developing its employees also helped alleviate the shortage of doctors and nurses by preparing staff to carry out tasks that previously required professional attention. (NOPH.)

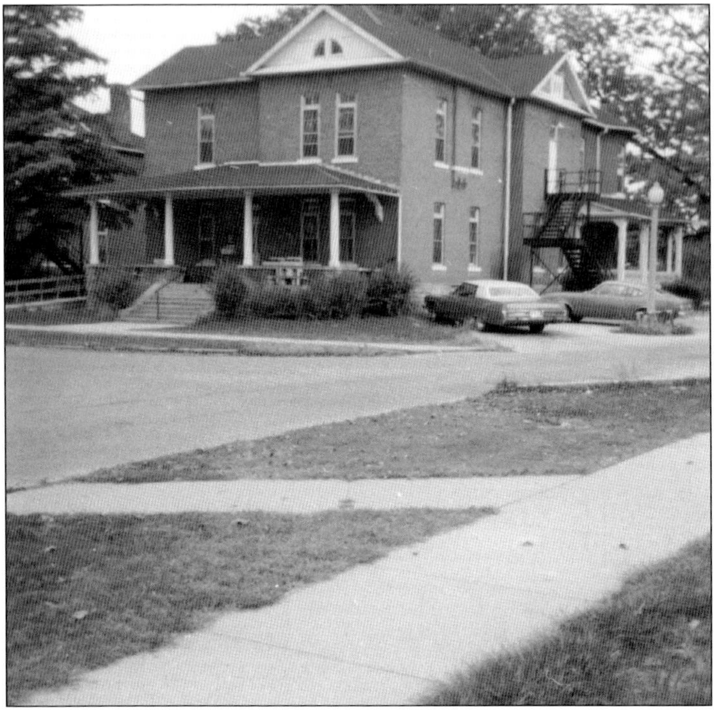

The Bureau of Vocational Rehabilitation was located in Cottage E at this time. A counselor there helped patients build resumes and learn job search techniques, and also worked with employers on placing former patients in jobs that matched their skills. Patients were also taught personal financial management in vocational rehabilitation. (NOPH.)

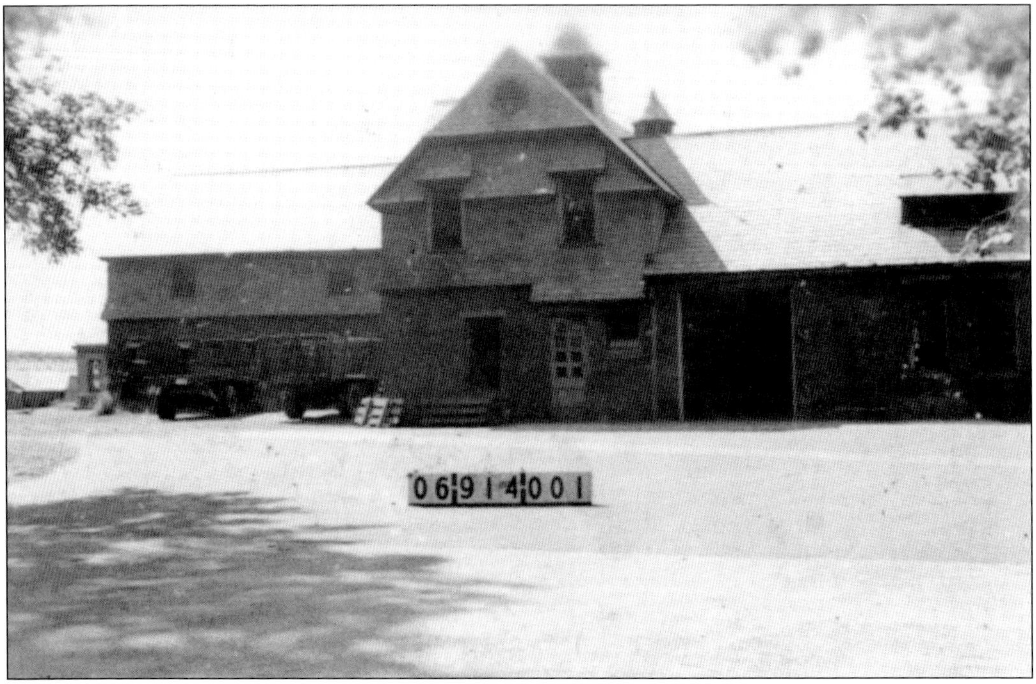

Ohio governor Michael DiSalle began phasing out all farming operations at the state hospitals in 1960, believing that they had become obsolete. In 1962, Toledo's dairy operation was discontinued, and the herd was transferred to the correctional facility at Massillon. The loss of jobs had a profound effect on the patient farmworkers. Productive work and their sense of self-worth, so important to their therapy, were taken away. (TLCPL.)

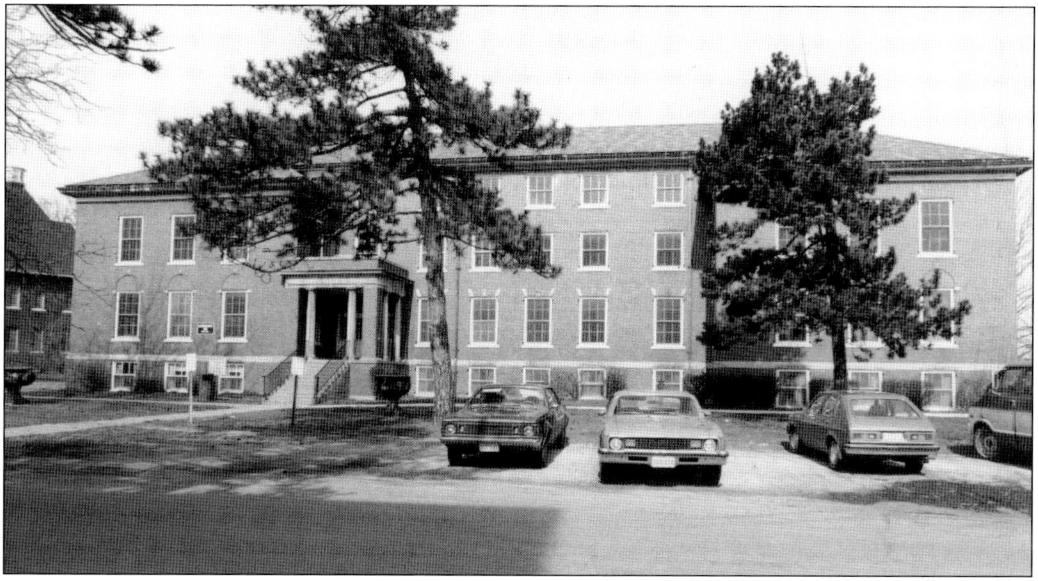

From the mid-1950s forward, several factors contributed to the decline in patient population at the hospital. By far, the biggest factor was that new and improved tranquilizing drugs became available and came into regular use. The hospital also expanded its social service programs and increased its professional medical staff. As a result, many patients improved so much that they were able to go home.

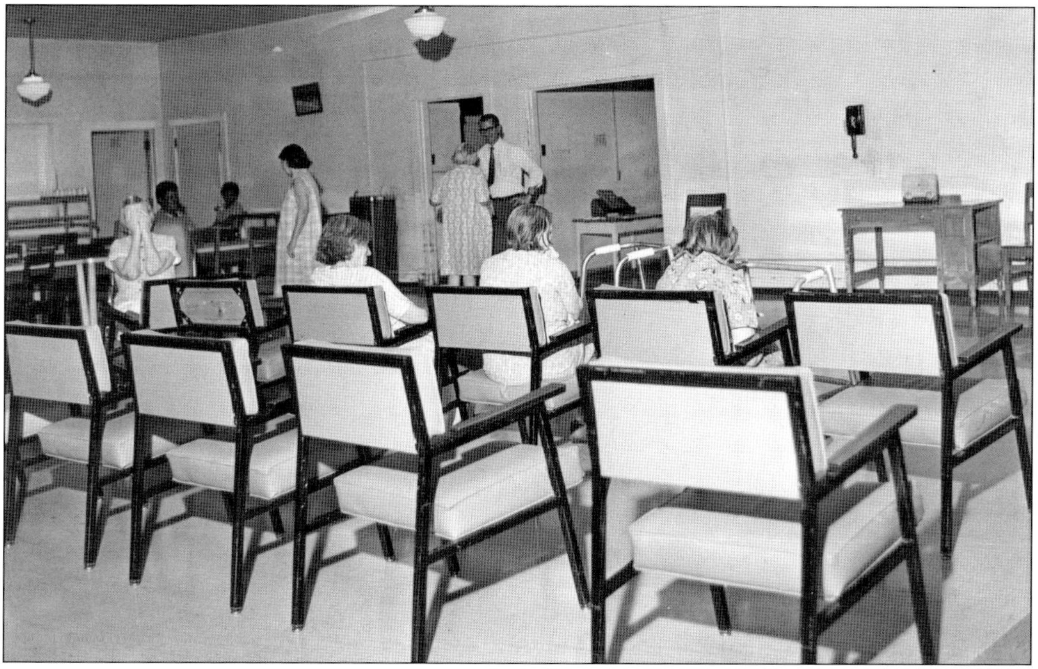

In 1960, Governor DiSalle began an effort to reduce overcrowding of the state's hospitals by transferring patients over the age of 65 to private nursing homes. He believed that state facilities had become a dumping ground for the aged—20 percent of Toledo's hospital population was aged 60 and over—and that while the elderly needed care, they did not need custodial psychiatric care. (NOPH.)

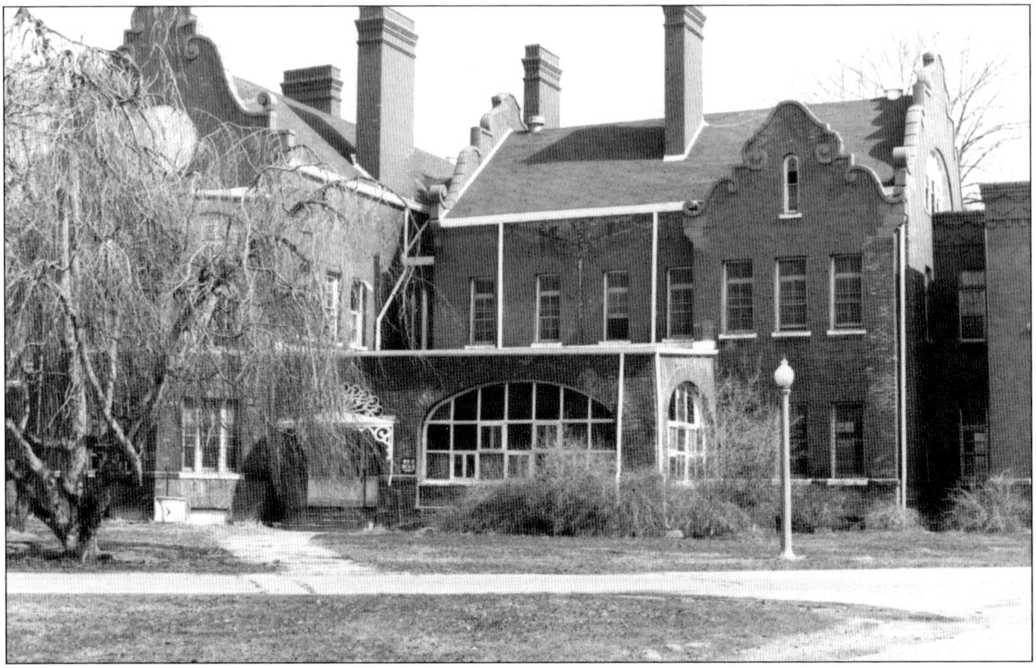

Pres. John F. Kennedy's Community Mental Health Act of 1963 changed the way mental health services were delivered from institutional-based care to community-based care. Federal dollars previously available to the state were diverted to the counties, and this led to a vast increase in the availability of mental health services in their communities. The act also emphasized prevention and supported research into the causes of mental illness and its treatment. (NOPH.)

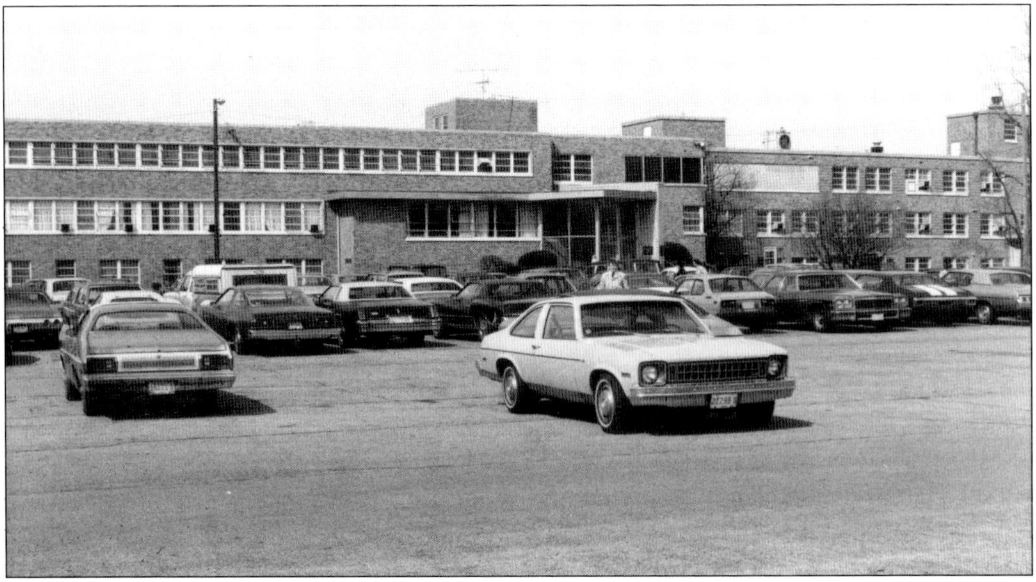

The hospital also increased its outpatient services. By the mid-1960s, it operated clinics in Lima, Defiance, Sandusky, and Toledo, as well as at the Receiving Hospital. These clinics were available to help patients transition from hospital life back into their communities. The Toledo District Nurses Association also provided nurses to visit patients who needed continued care after returning home. (TLCPL.)

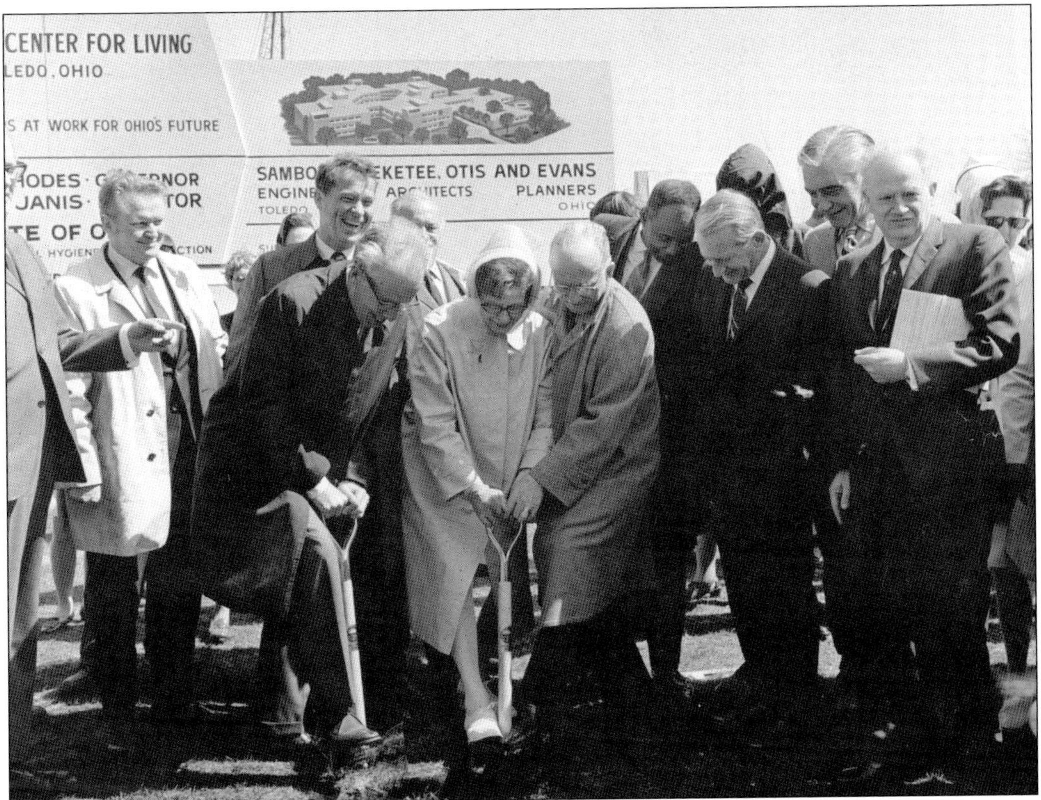

By 1970, those not needing inpatient care were released to group homes, nursing homes, and to their families, continuing treatment in outpatient and community clinics. The population, which had peaked at over 3,000 in 1955, steadily dwindled to around 300. Those remaining were transferred to the newer buildings. Also this year, ground was broken for the new Geriatric Building, which would replace Cottage 14 and Cottage 12. (NOPH.)

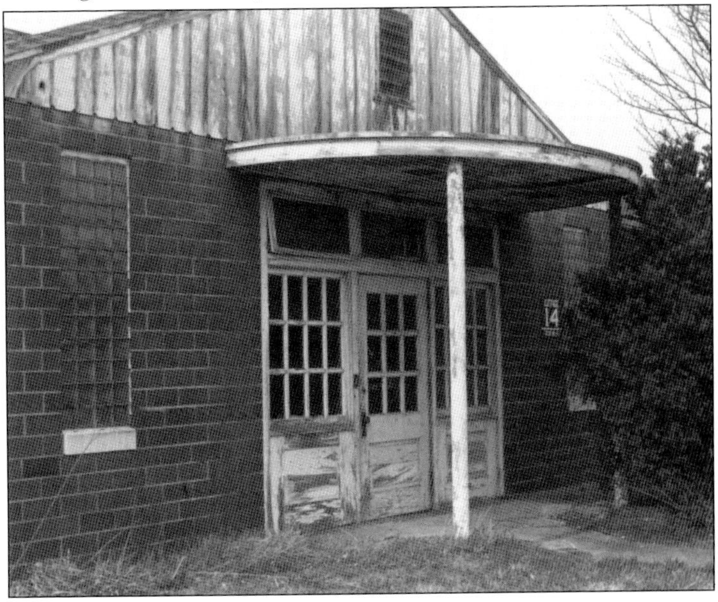

At the same time that the patient population was declining, the condition of the hospital's physical structures continued to decline as well, and many had become unsafe. Throughout the 1960s and into the 1970s, as the buildings were emptied, they were razed. Most were gone by 1980. This photograph shows the condition of Cottage 14 in 1976. (NOPH.)

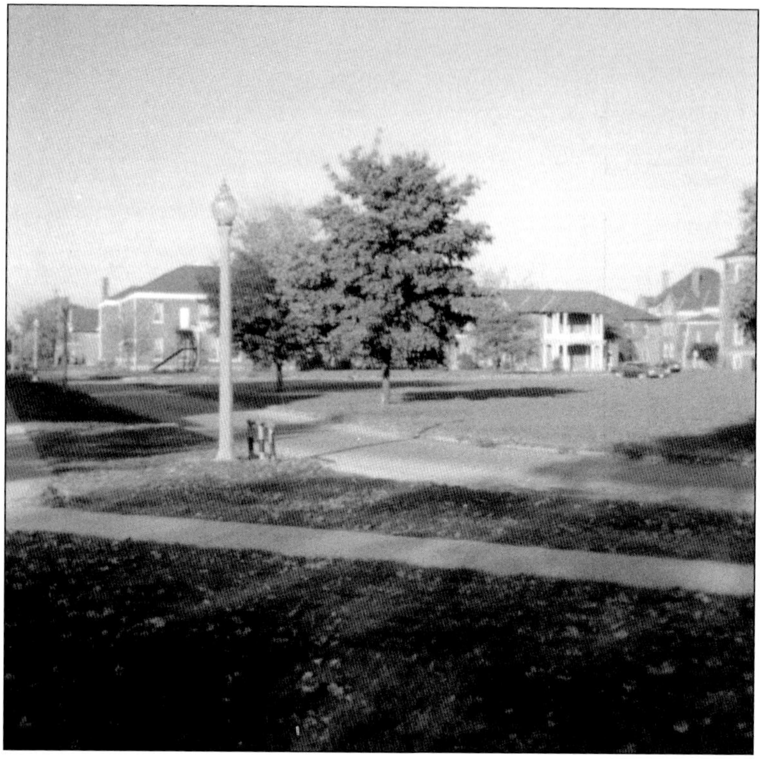

This is a view of the south end of the hospital grounds in 1976. From left to right are the old firehouse, Food Service Building, Industrial Building, Female Hall, Administration Building, the post office, and a portion of the Nurses Home. All of them would be gone by 1980. (NOPH.)

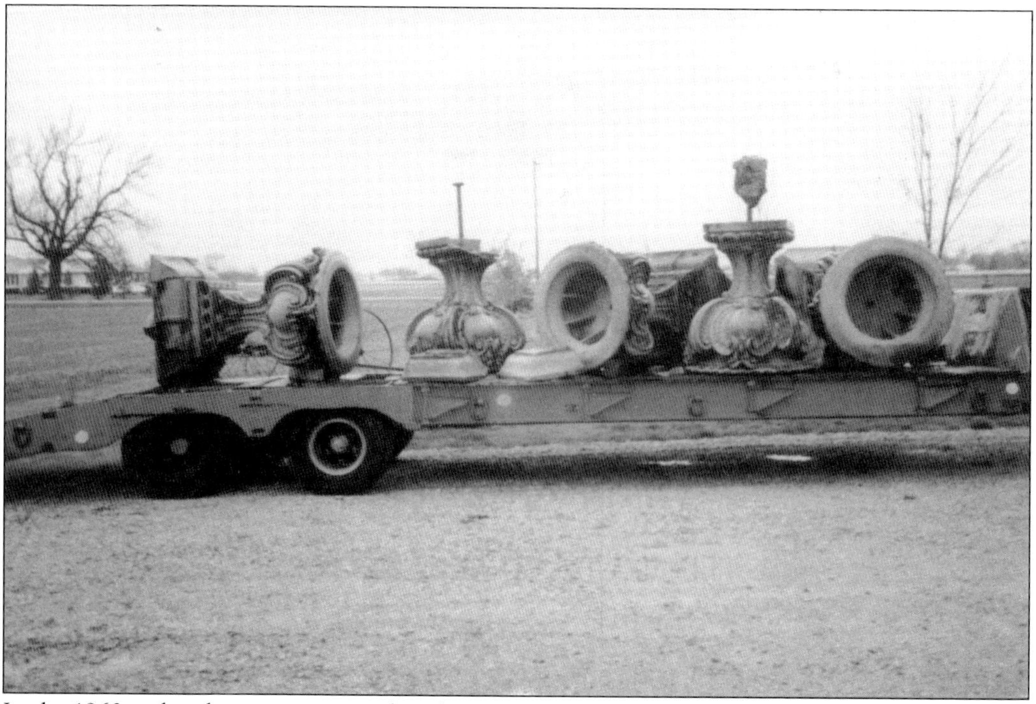

In the 1960s, a local tree service was hired to remove trees, sidewalks, other landscaping features, and to destroy and remove the many beautiful terra cotta planting urns that decorated the grounds. The owner of the company recognized their beauty and value and salvaged five of them. (NOPH.)

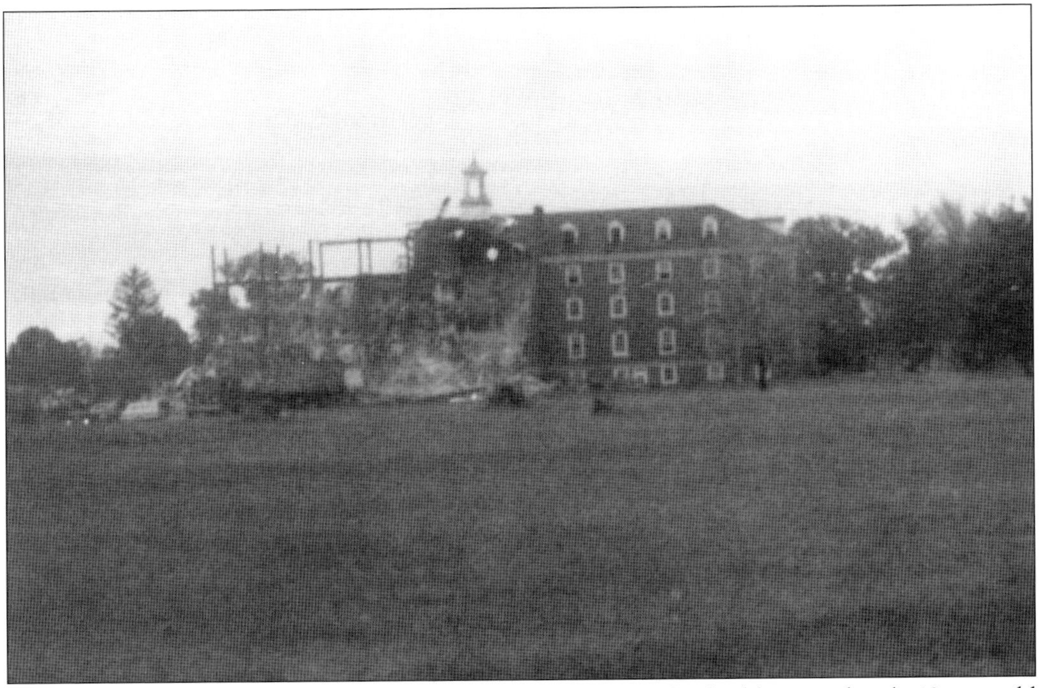

This photograph shows the Nurses Home during demolition. This building was barely 40 years old and was still in good condition when it was torn down. Photographs show that it had beautiful fixtures, ornate transom windows, and solid wood paneling and doors. (NOPH.)

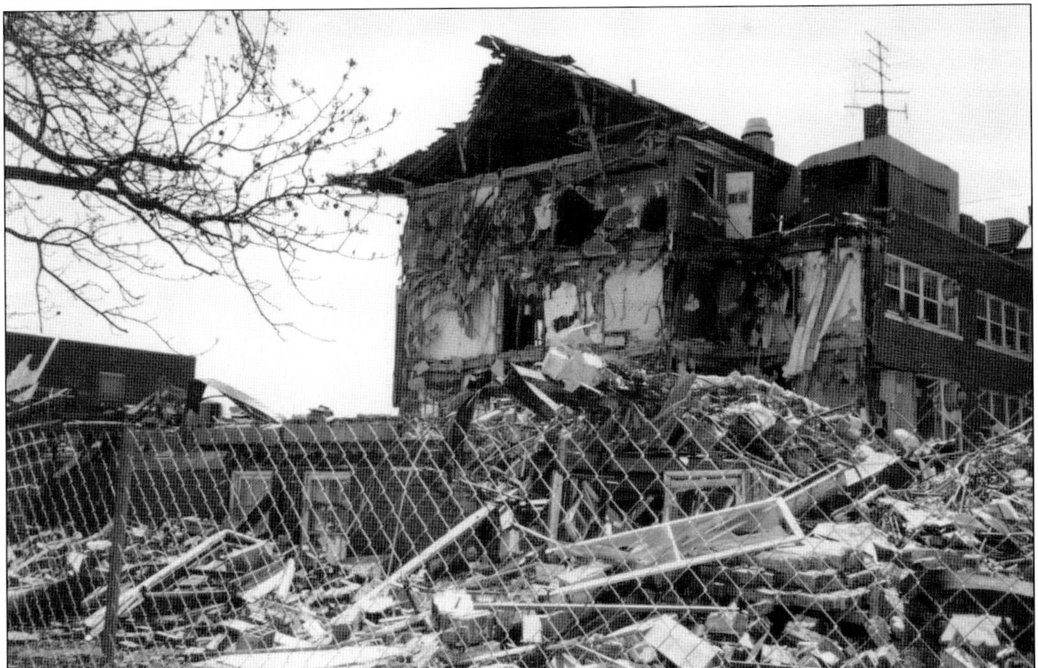

This is the rear of the Neuropsychiatric Building during demolition. Built in 1930, it was first known as WH6/MH5 Medical and Surgical and later as Building 1 for the chronically medically ill. (NOPH.)

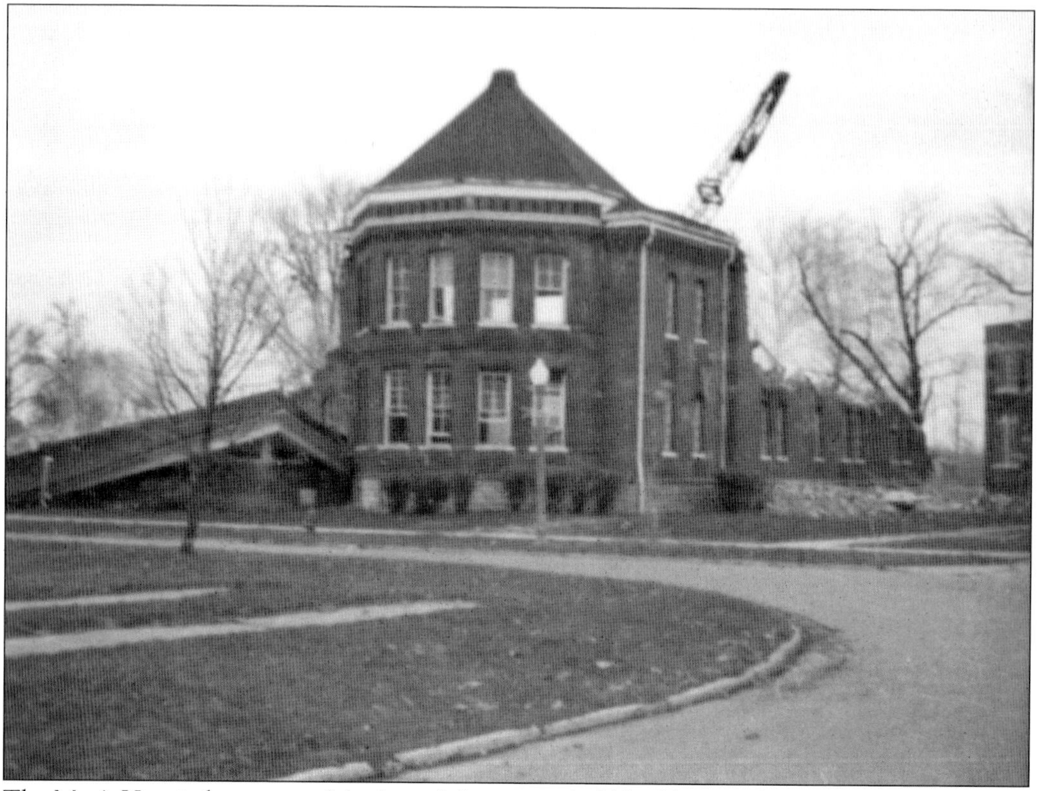

The Men's Hospital was one of the last of the original old buildings to be torn down. The Men's Hospital, Women's Hospital, and chapel were all destroyed in 1981. (NOPH.)

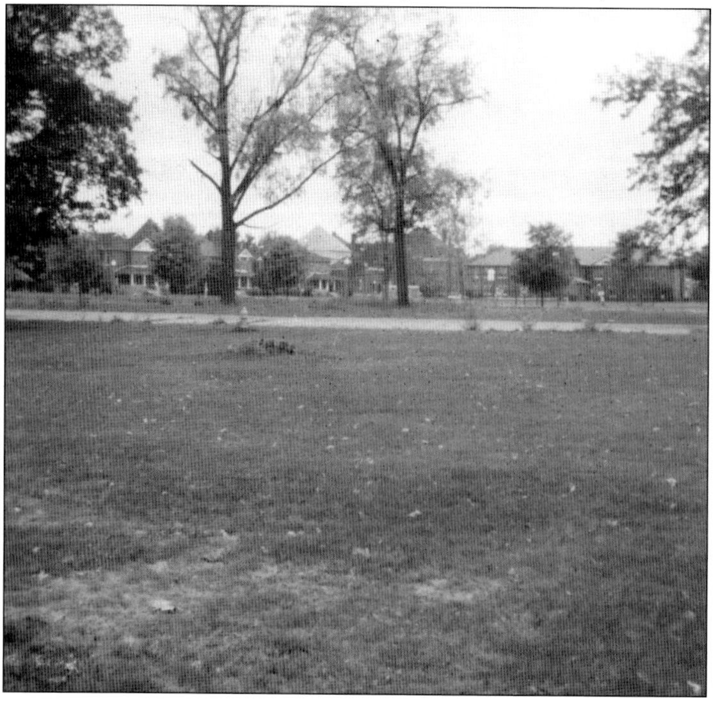

Taken from the site where Cottage 10 once stood, this photograph looks across the former recreation field to Cottages 3, 2, and 1, and the Entertainment Hall. Fred Bigelow, former hospital business manager, photographed all of the buildings still standing in 1976, just prior to their destruction. (NOPH.)

The last religious service was held in the chapel in 1978. The sharp decline in patient population had had an impact on the Catholic ministry at the hospital, and attendance at weekly services was down from an average of 220 to 35. The building was closed after this service and was demolished in 1981. Its stained-glass windows, including its "rose window," had been missing since before 1969. (NOPH.)

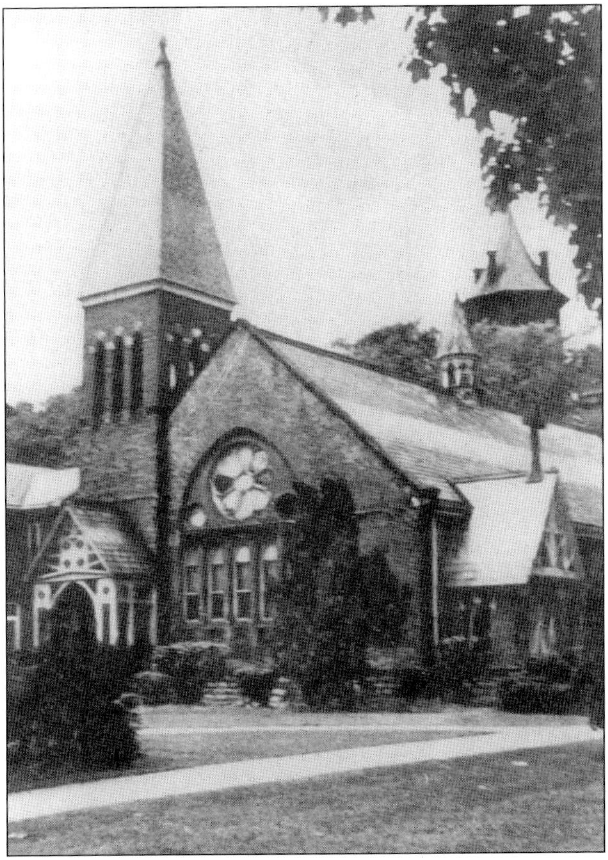

In 1971, the hospital's name was changed to Toledo Mental Health Center, and in 1998, it became the Northcoast Behavioral Healthcare–Toledo Campus. Today, the Northwest Ohio Psychiatric Hospital operates on the site and provides mental healthcare, addiction treatment, and prevention services to Toledo and the surrounding area. (NOPH.)

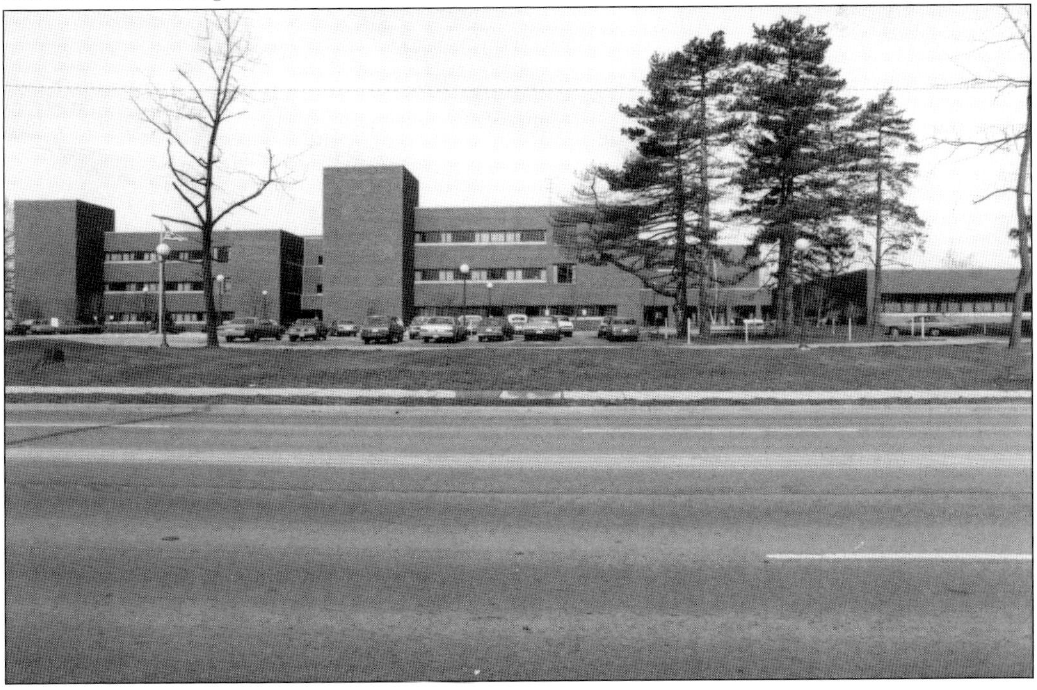

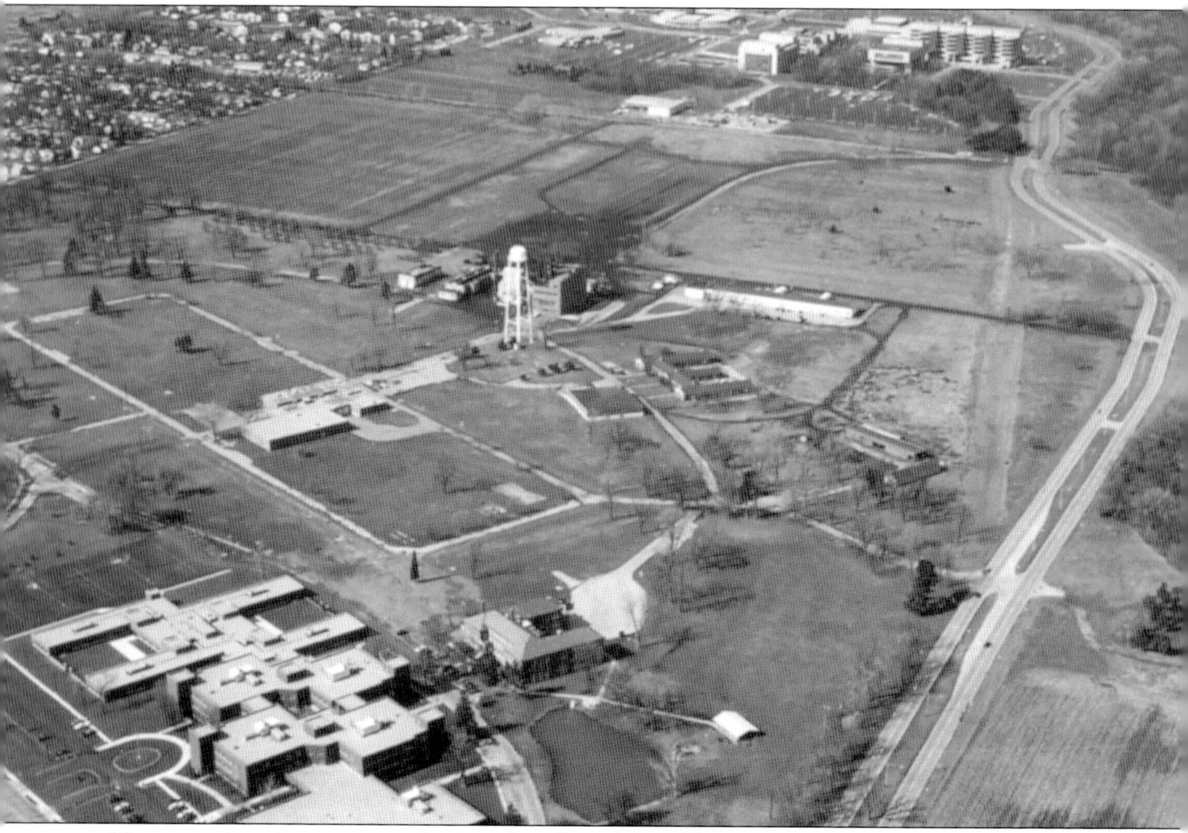

The sweeping changes over the last decades of the old hospital had made provisions for some, but not for all. Many patients slipped through the cracks and did not receive the care that they needed. They were discharged to the street, with nowhere to go and without the wherewithal to follow through with treatment. Unable to care for themselves, they were left to wander, just like they did hundreds of years ago. (NOPH.)

Six

The Cemeteries

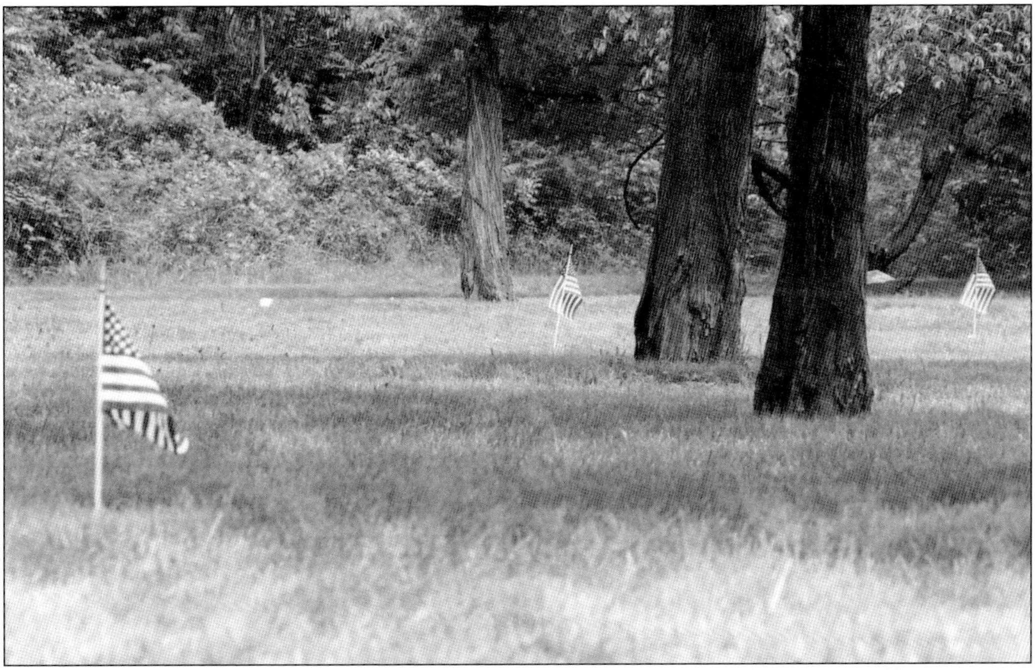

Those who came to the hospital for help did so at a time when mental illness was still very much a mystery, and treatment methods, even the successful ones, were not understood. Sometimes they recovered and returned to their families and communities. Many did not and spent the remainder of their lives as patients. Those who died there and whose bodies were not claimed were buried in one of the hospital's two cemeteries. (NOPH.)

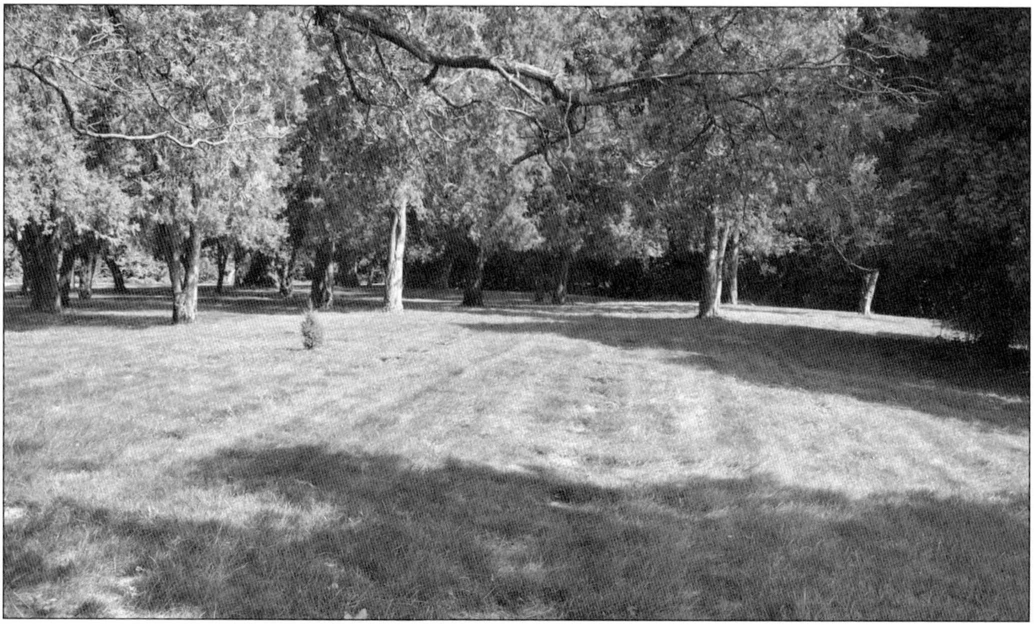

In the two cemeteries on the hospital grounds are the graves of 1,994 patients whose bodies were unclaimed by family or friends. The first documented burial was in June 1888. The last was November 17, 1973. Until recently, the only physical evidence indicating the existence of the cemeteries were depressions in the ground and tiny grave markers, many of which had sunken and were no longer visible. (Photograph by author.)

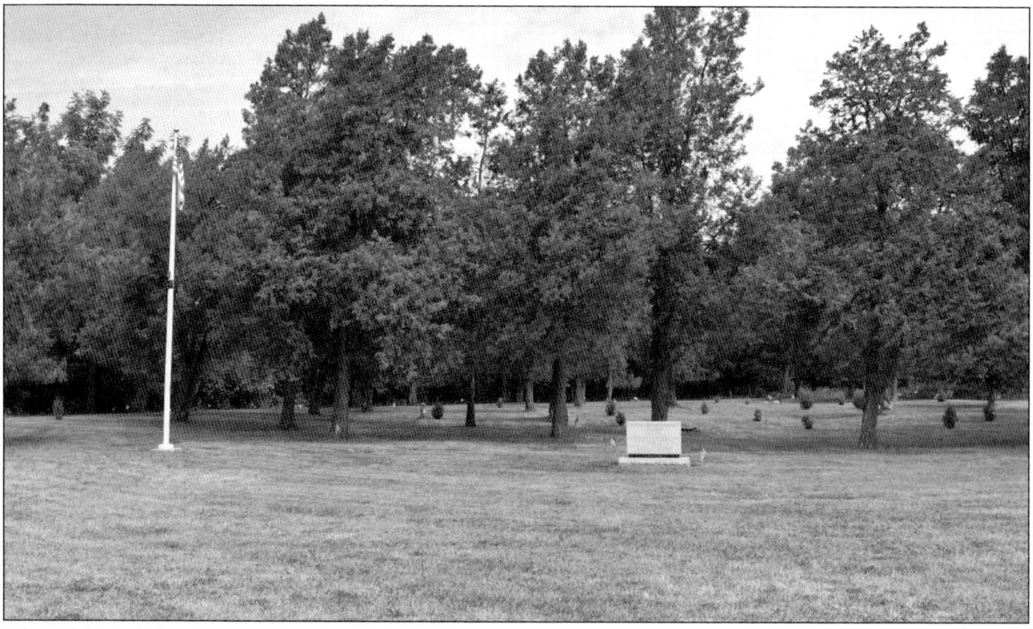

The older of the two cemeteries, located on Arlington Avenue, contains over 900 graves and was used from 1888 until 1922. For a time, the hospital farm's pig runs were located immediately adjacent to it. This cemetery is bordered by Swan Creek, and today, one can find refuse from the hospital on the creek bank, indicating that it was, for some time, part of a trash dump. (Photograph by author.)

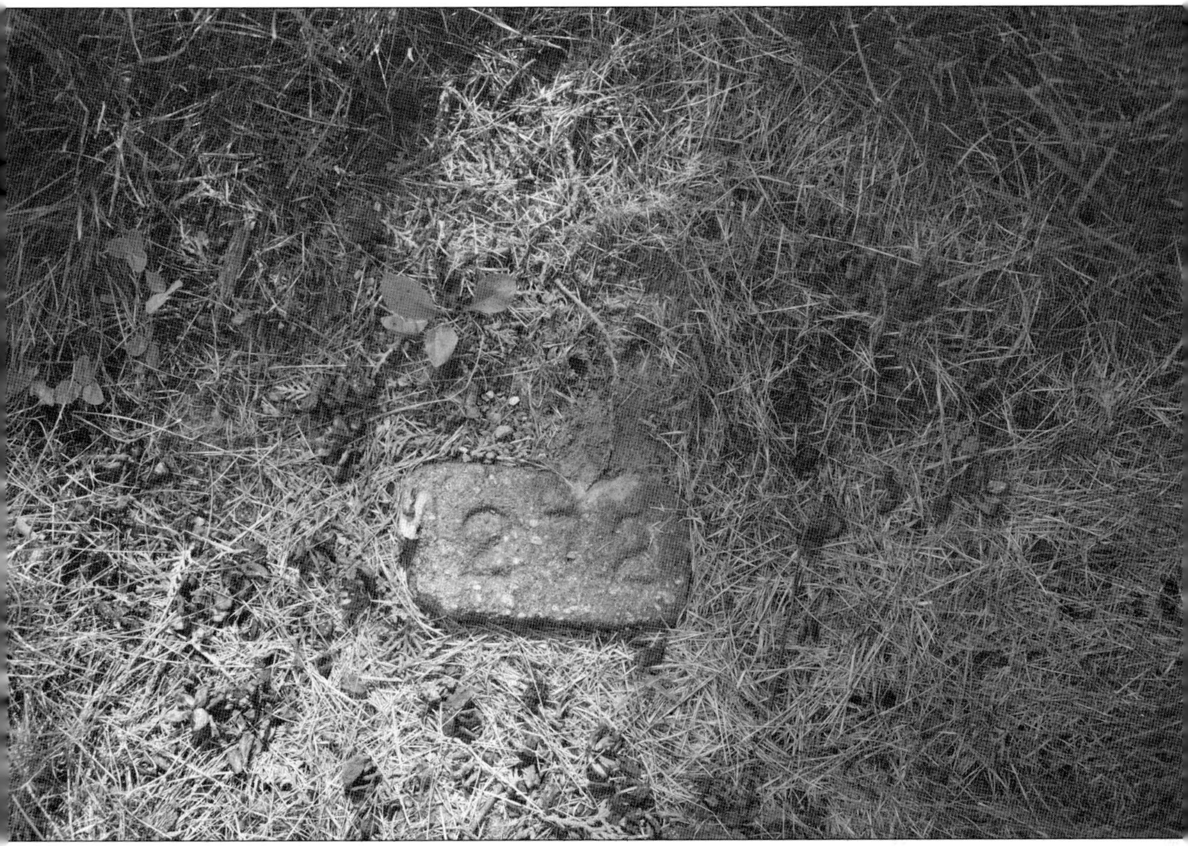

The graves in the cemeteries are marked only with tiny, numbered concrete blocks that were manufactured by patients at the hospital. The numbers correspond to names in the hospital's burial log books. Many of the markers have sunken into the ground due to the shifting of the earth over time and due to neglect. (Photograph by author.)

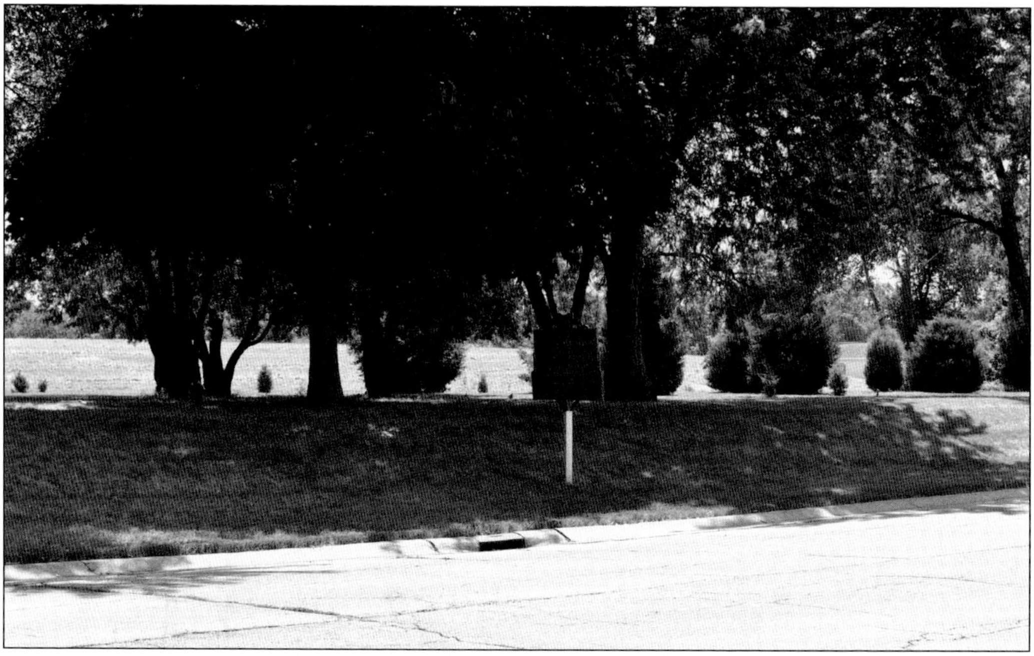

The newer of the two cemeteries is located on East Medical Loop Drive on the University of Toledo's Health Science Campus and was used from 1922 to 1973. It contains the graves of over 1,100 people. Over the years, thousands of students have driven by and attended classes directly across the street, completely unaware that it was there. (Photograph by author.)

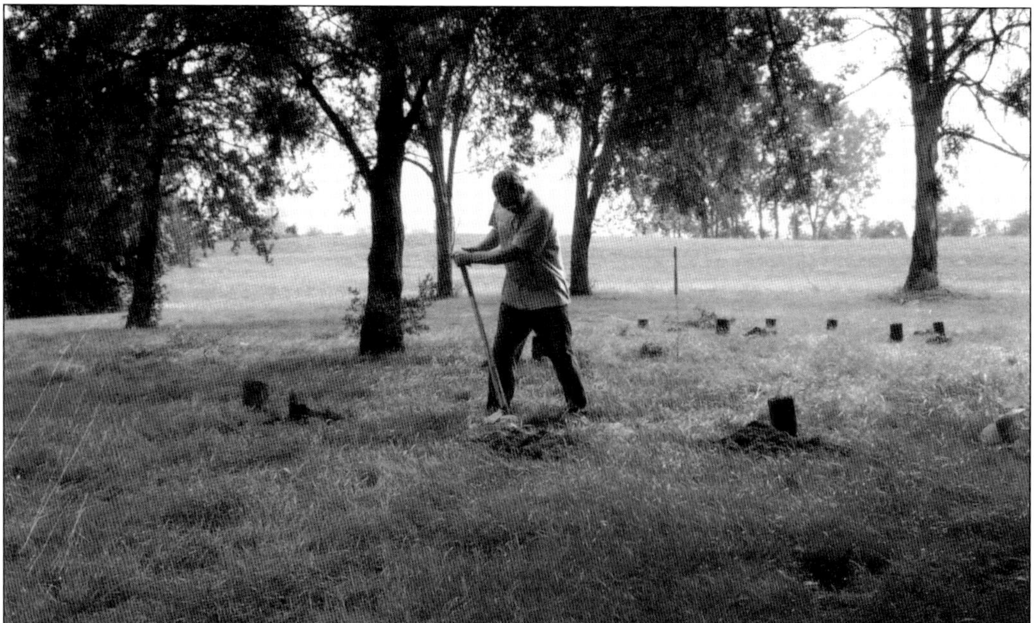

In 2005, the Toledo State Hospital Cemetery Reclamation Project (TSHCRP) was organized. Here, a volunteer member works to locate and raise small grave markers that have sunken into the earth over time. Since the committee's work began, approximately 1,364 markers have been found and raised, but hundreds more remain lost. (NOPH.)

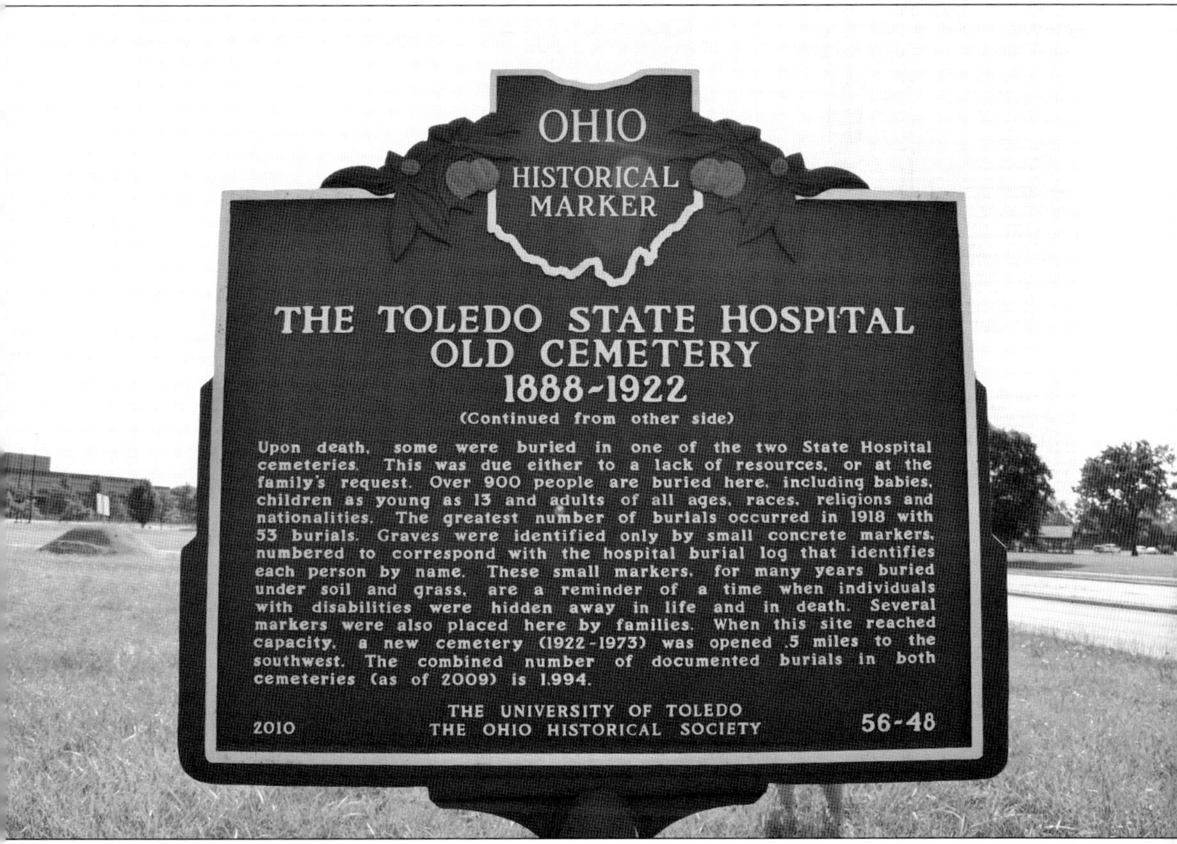
OHIO
HISTORICAL
MARKER
THE TOLEDO STATE HOSPITAL
OLD CEMETERY
1888-1922
(Continued from other side)
Upon death, some were buried in one of the two State Hospital cemeteries. This was due either to a lack of resources, or at the family's request. Over 900 people are buried here, including babies, children as young as 13 and adults of all ages, races, religions and nationalities. The greatest number of burials occurred in 1918 with 53 burials. Graves were identified only by small concrete markers, numbered to correspond with the hospital burial log that identifies each person by name. These small markers, for many years buried under soil and grass, are a reminder of a time when individuals with disabilities were hidden away in life and in death. Several markers were also placed here by families. When this site reached capacity, a new cemetery (1922-1973) was opened .5 miles to the southwest. The combined number of documented burials in both cemeteries (as of 2009) is 1,994.
2010
THE UNIVERSITY OF TOLEDO
THE OHIO HISTORICAL SOCIETY
56-48

Thanks to the work of the Cemetery Reclamation Project, Ohio Historical Society markers have been installed in both cemeteries and are situated in places visible to passersby. This one stands next to Arlington Avenue at the Old Cemetery. (Photograph by author.)

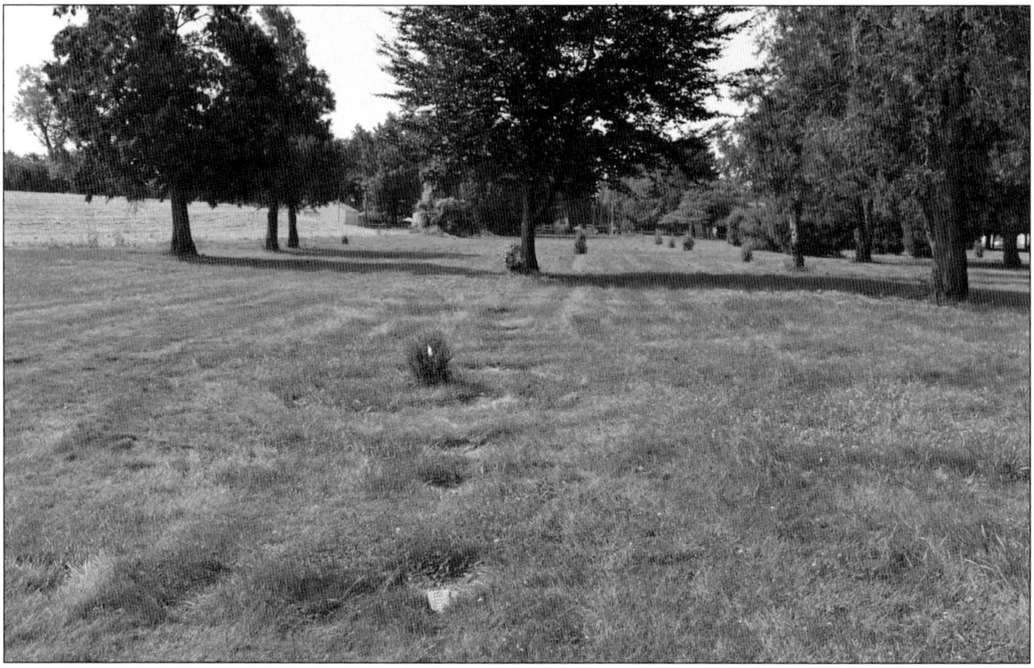

Looking across the burial field that is the New Cemetery, it is difficult to realize even now that it is a cemetery. While much work has been done to mark the cemeteries and locate and uncover the individual grave markers, they are tiny and are quickly covered over again with cut grass and fallen leaves. (Photograph by author.)

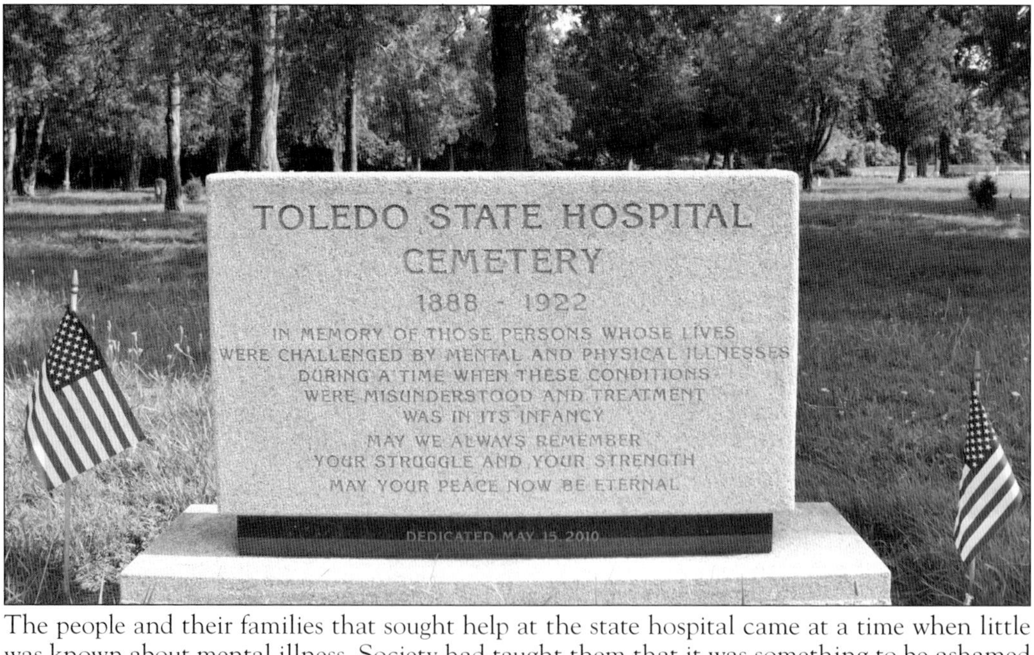
TOLEDO STATE HOSPITAL
CEMETERY
1888 - 1922
IN MEMORY OF THOSE PERSONS WHOSE LIVES
WERE CHALLENGED BY MENTAL AND PHYSICAL ILLNESSES
DURING A TIME WHEN THESE CONDITIONS
WERE MISUNDERSTOOD AND TREATMENT
WAS IN ITS INFANCY
MAY WE ALWAYS REMEMBER
YOUR STRUGGLE AND YOUR STRENGTH
MAY YOUR PEACE NOW BE ETERNAL
DEDICATED MAY 15, 2010

The people and their families that sought help at the state hospital came at a time when little was known about mental illness. Society had taught them that it was something to be ashamed of—something to be hidden. This granite monument now stands at the entrance to the Old Cemetery. Its few words reflect this and set a solemn and respectful tone for the visitor. (Photograph by author.)

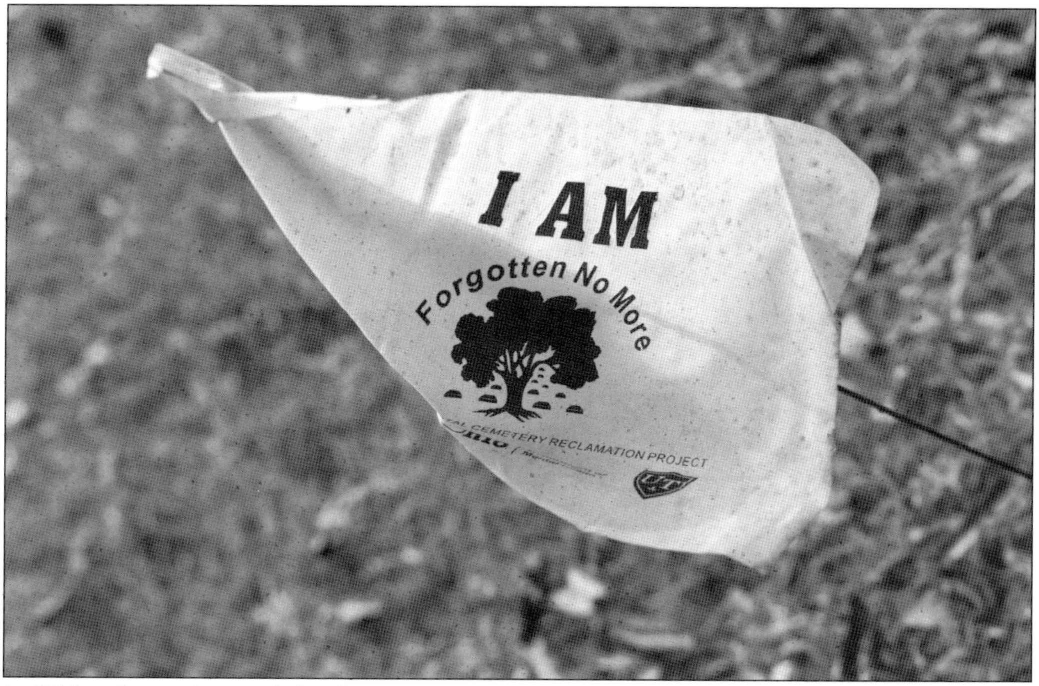

In 2010, a former hospital chaplain remembered that sometimes families would bring their ill to the hospital and then forget about them. He spoke of the sadness he felt when conducting a funeral that no one showed up for. Every spring, Cemetery Reclamation Project volunteers decorate each grave with a flag that reads, "I am forgotten no more." (Photograph by author.)

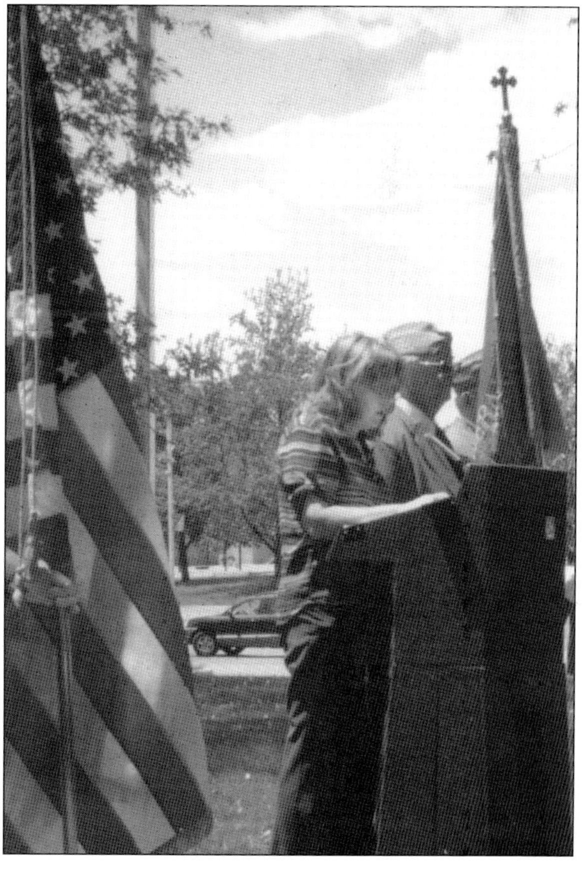

Each year on Armed Forces Day, the TSHCRP hosts a memorial service in the cemeteries to remember those who were forgotten in life. Various veterans' organizations participate and place wreaths in each of the cemeteries to honor the veterans who are buried there. Jane Graham Weber, chairperson of the project, is shown here at the podium. (NOPH.)

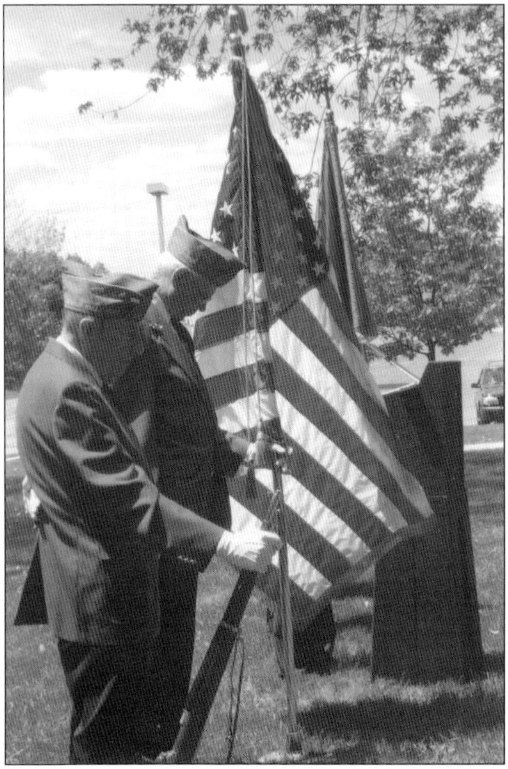

Although the annual memorial service is meant to remember all of those buried in the cemeteries, various veterans' organizations have played a major role in the program each year. There are 77 known veterans in the cemeteries, and they represent every war from the Civil War to World War II. (NOPH.)

The cemeteries are a microcosm of the former hospital's community. Those buried in them represent all walks of life, all ethnicities, all religions, and all classes of society. They came for help and often spent decades of their lives there, only to be forgotten in life and then again in death. For years, the cemeteries went neglected and over time became invisible, just like the people who were buried in them. (NOPH.)

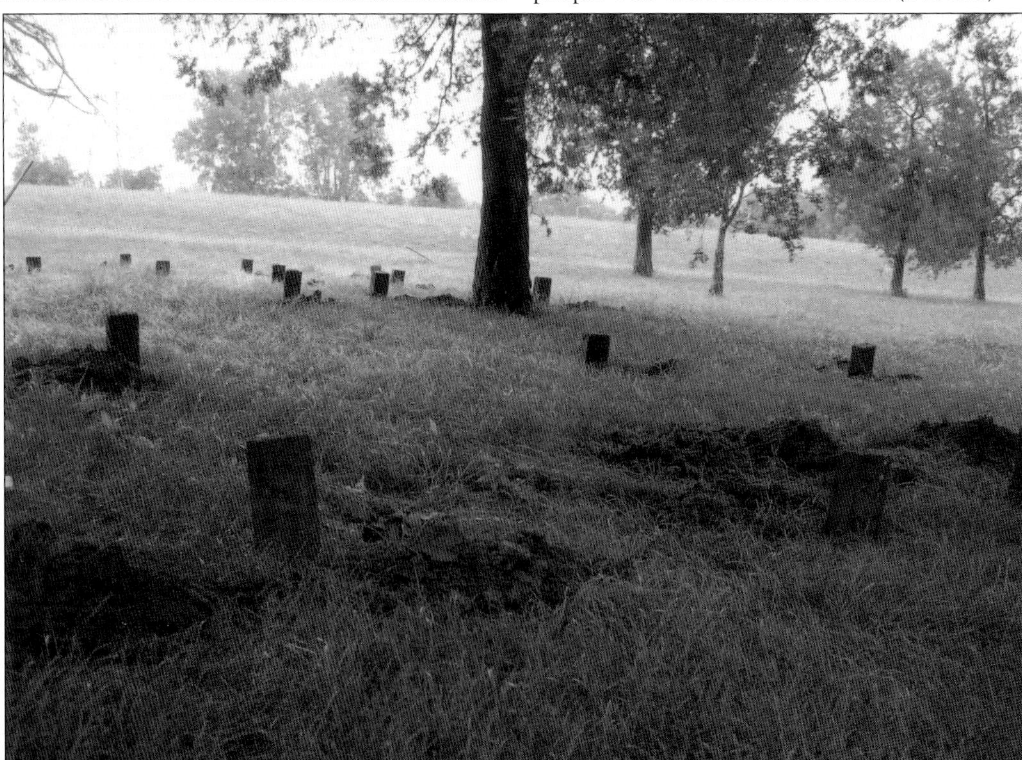

Seven

THEN AND NOW

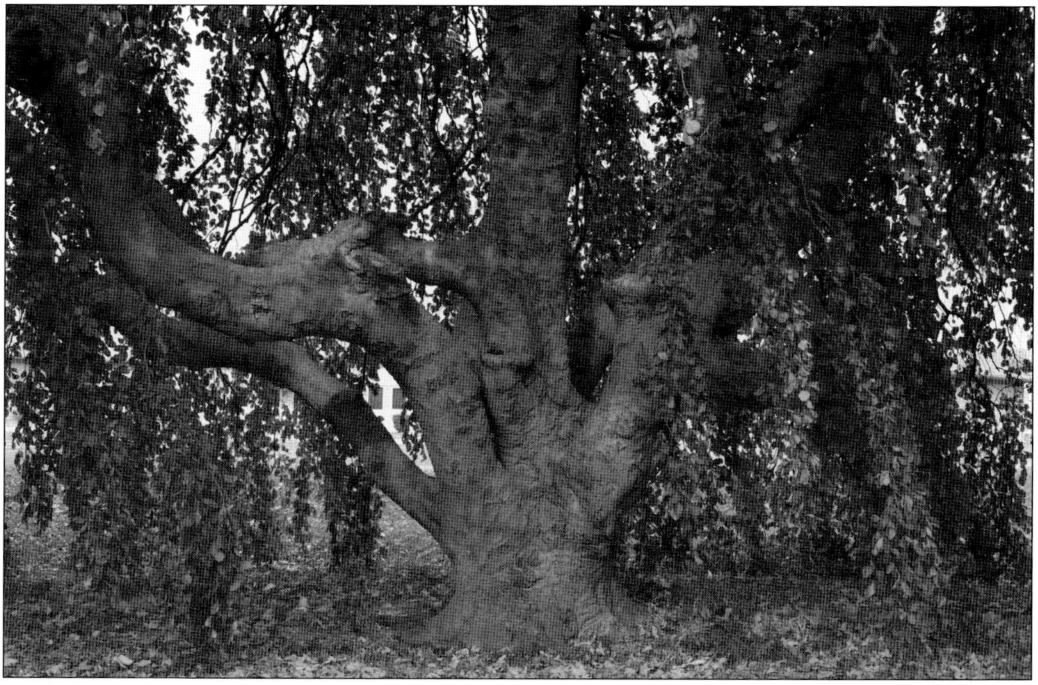

Aside from the cemeteries, very little that is tangible remains of the old state hospital today. This large old beech tree, scarred with carvings by patients, staff, and visitors, still stands and bears witness to their presence so long ago. It was known to local children as the "elephant tree" because of its bumpy skin. (Photograph by author.)

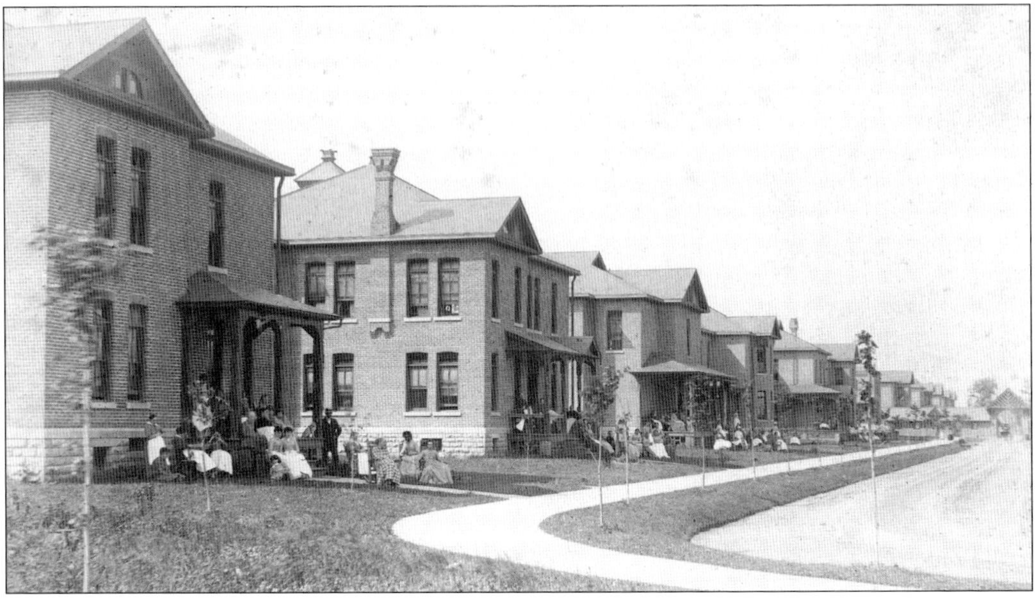

These photographs show a section of Inner Drive, the inner rectangle around the hospital campus that the cottages and other original buildings faced, around 1890, and what is left of it now. (Above, TLCPL; below, photograph by author.)

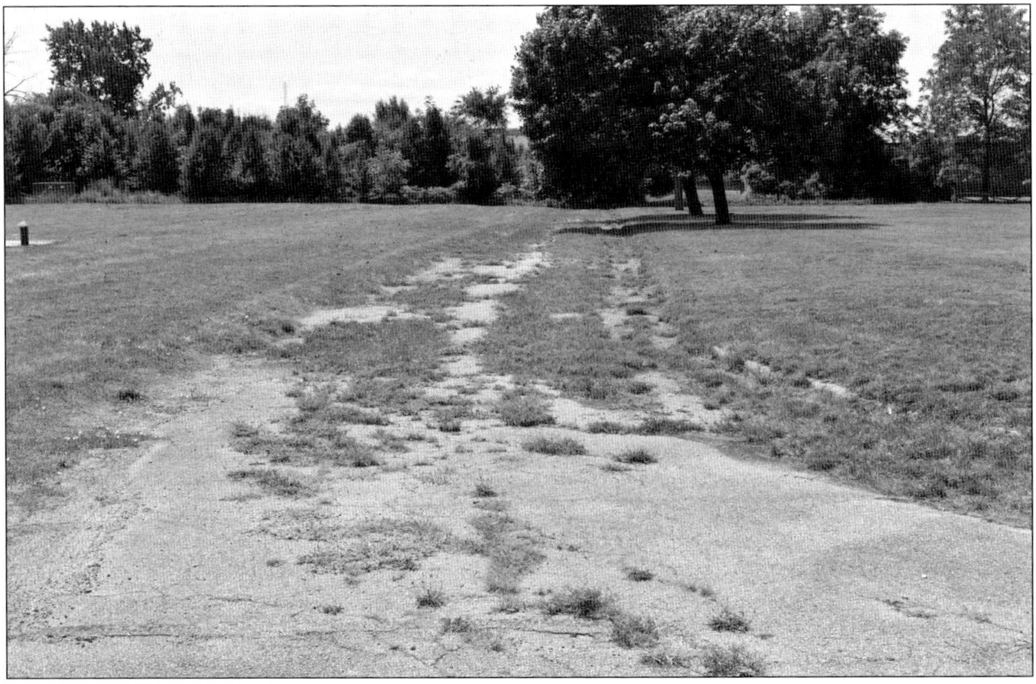

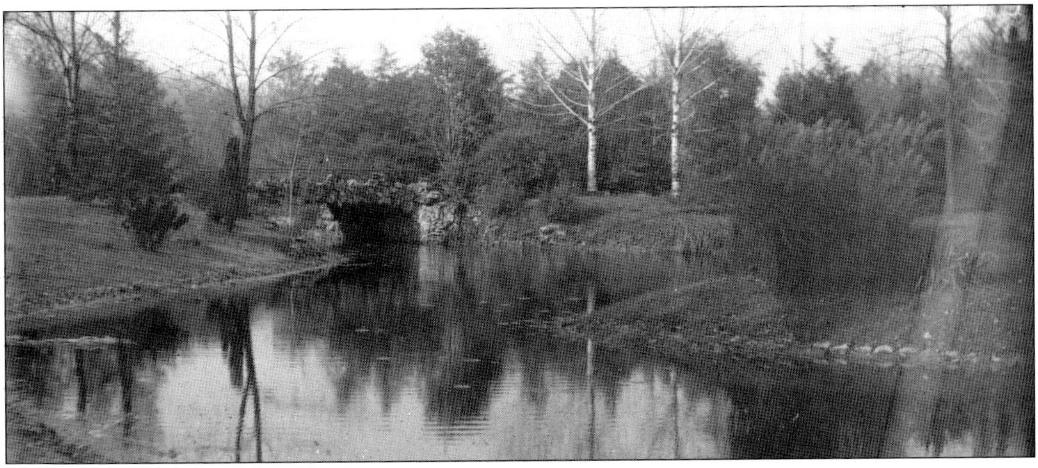

Four of the original lagoons still beautify the property. This one was considered part of the golf course and is distinguished by its small island. (Above, TLCPL; below, photograph by author.)

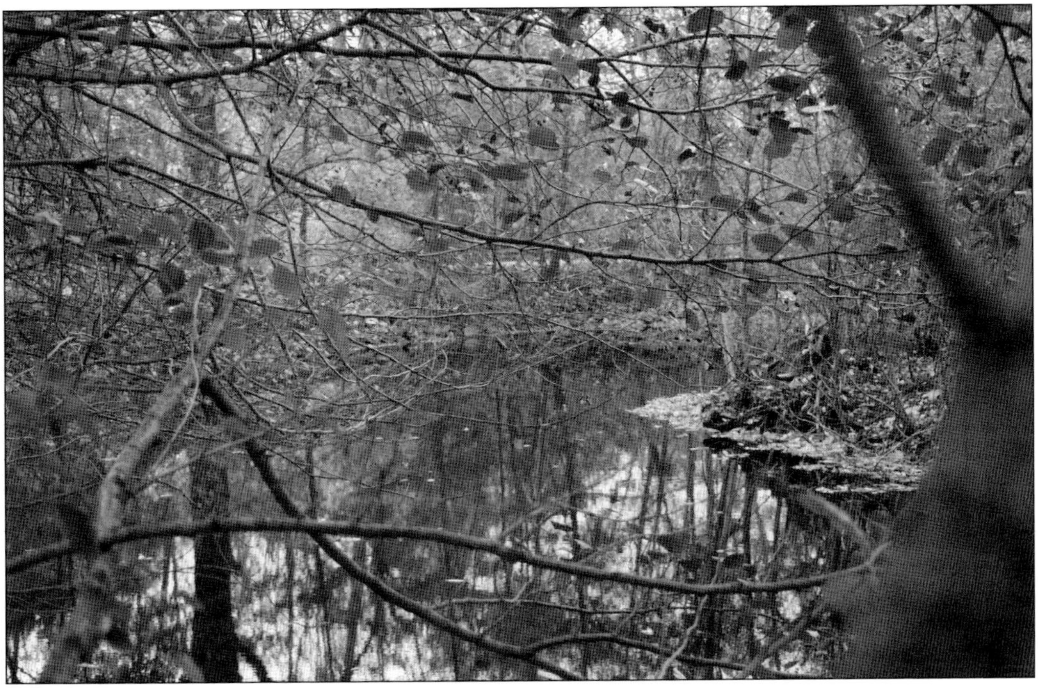

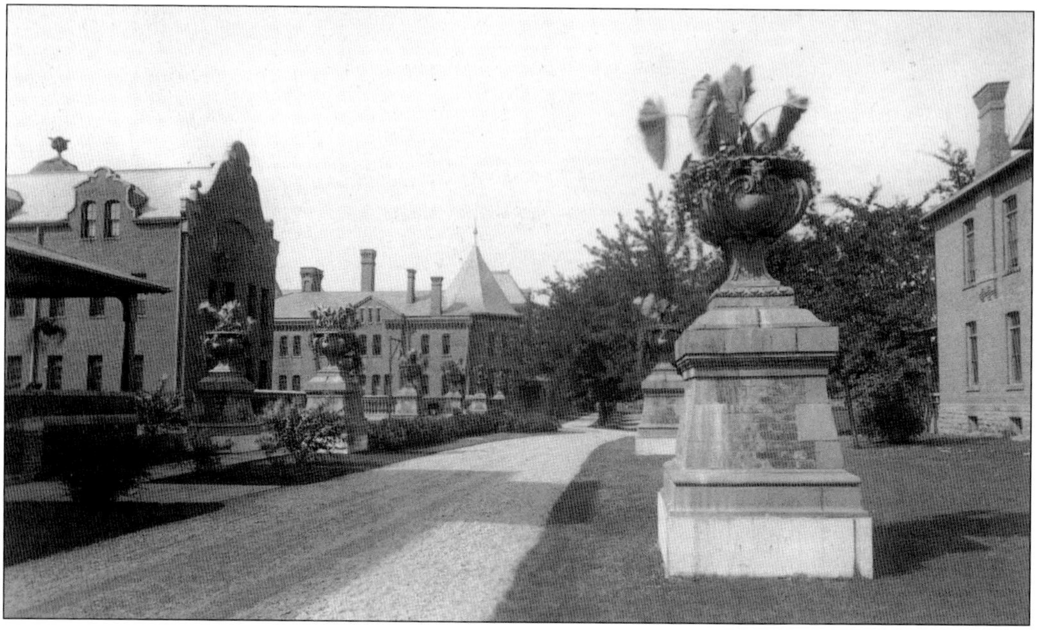

In the late 1960s, a local tree service was hired to destroy and remove the huge terra cotta urns that had graced the hospital grounds for nearly 100 years. The owner of the company, however, recognized their beauty and saved five of them, and in 1998, his daughters sold them at auction. One is now located in the Little Italy section of Cleveland, and the other four were purchased by an out of town buyer. Three more somehow survived and now decorate the entrance to the Northwest Ohio Psychiatric Hospital. (Above, NOPH; below, photograph by author.)

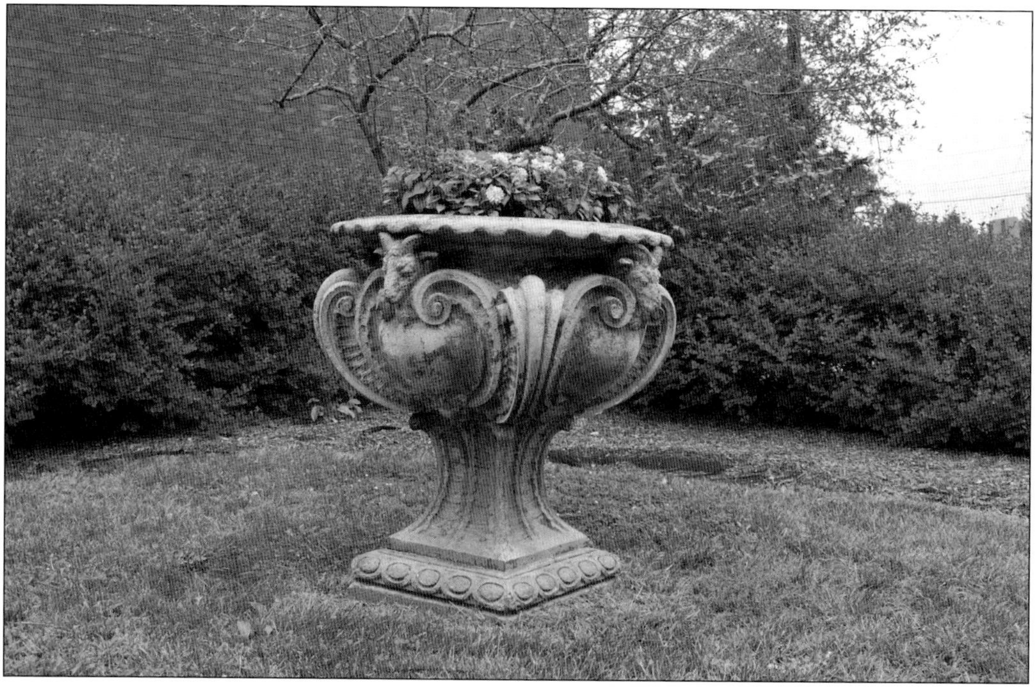

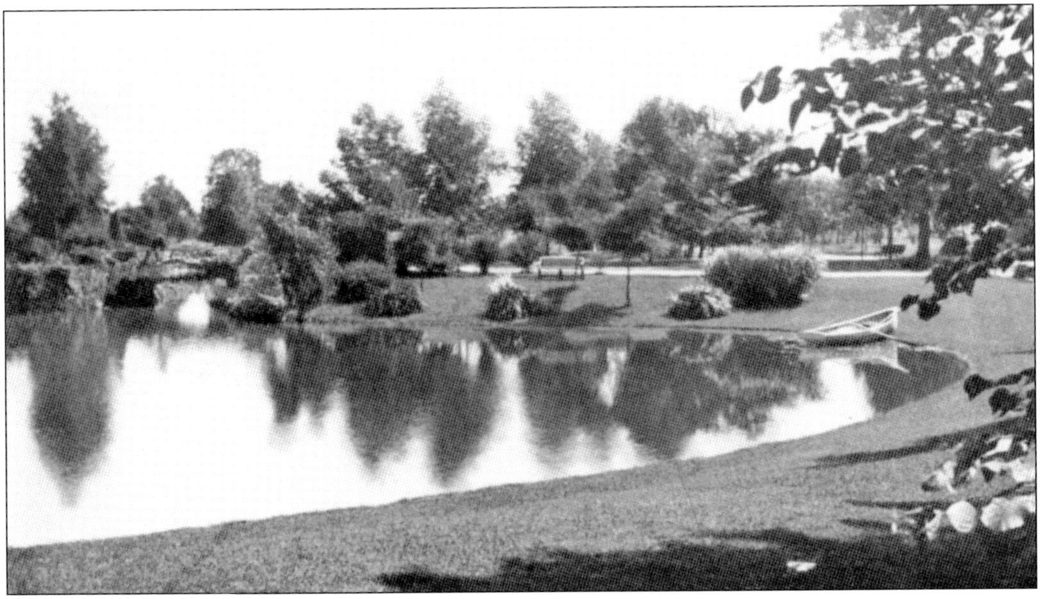

A later concrete footbridge between the two northern lagoons is in ruins now. (Above, NOPH; below, photograph by author.)

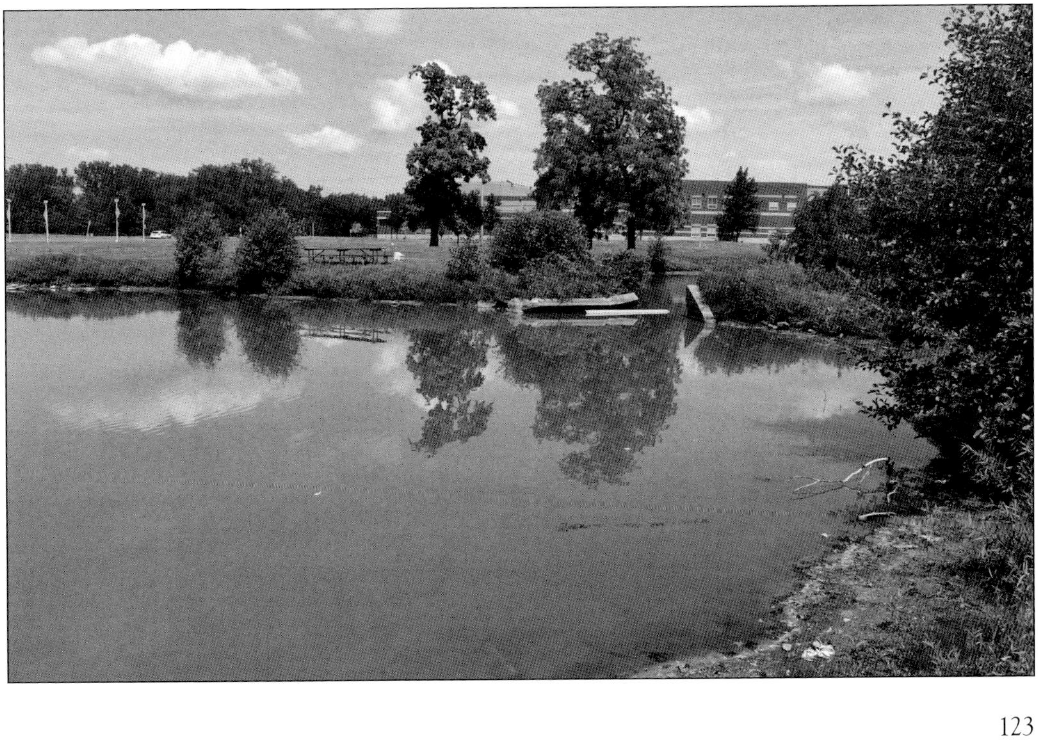

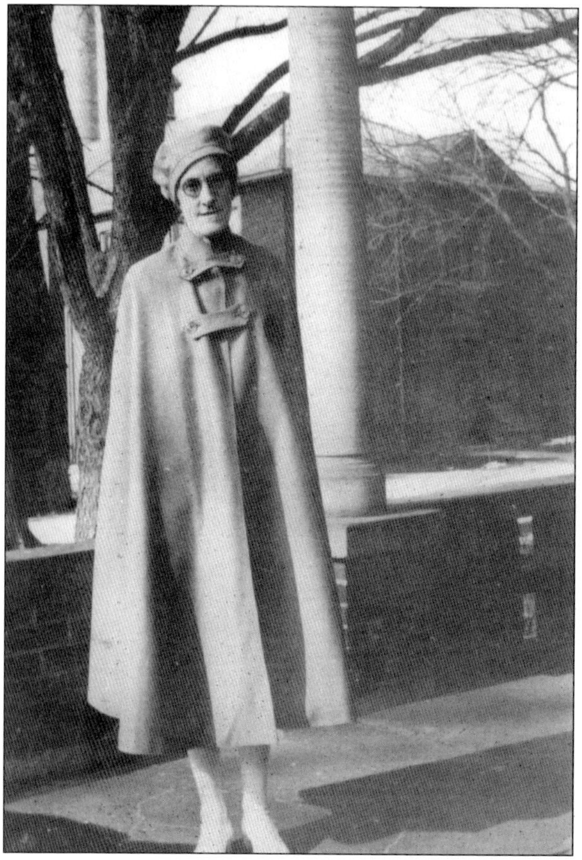

The cape on the mannequin below was donated to the Archives Room Museum at the Northwest Ohio Psychiatric Hospital. It is identical to the cape worn by the nurse in the c. 1930 photograph to the left. (Left, NOPH; below, photograph by author.)

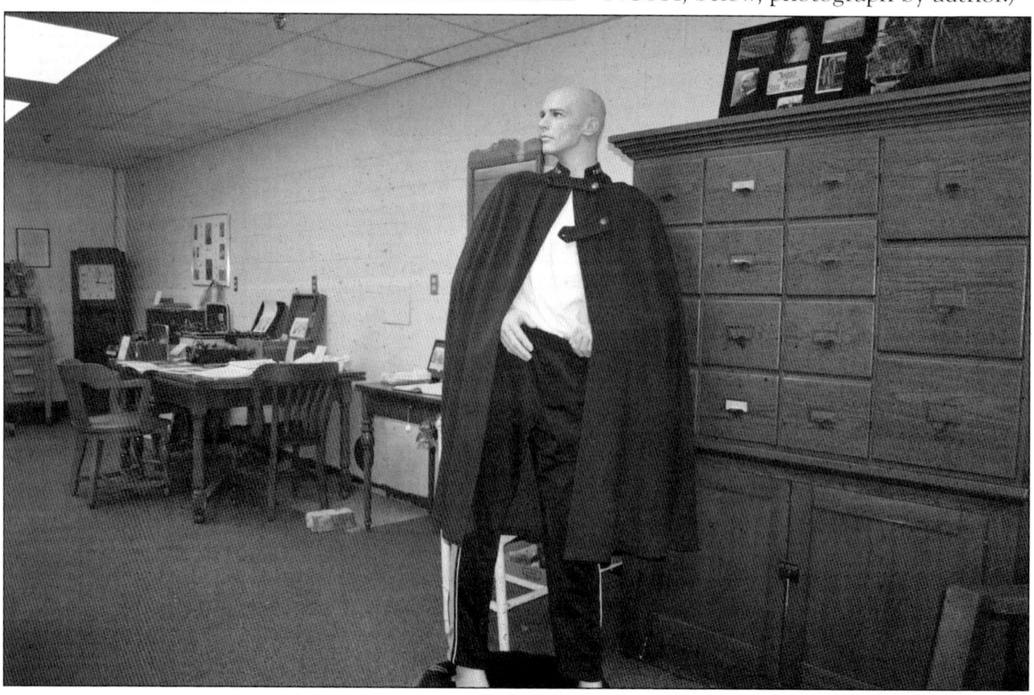

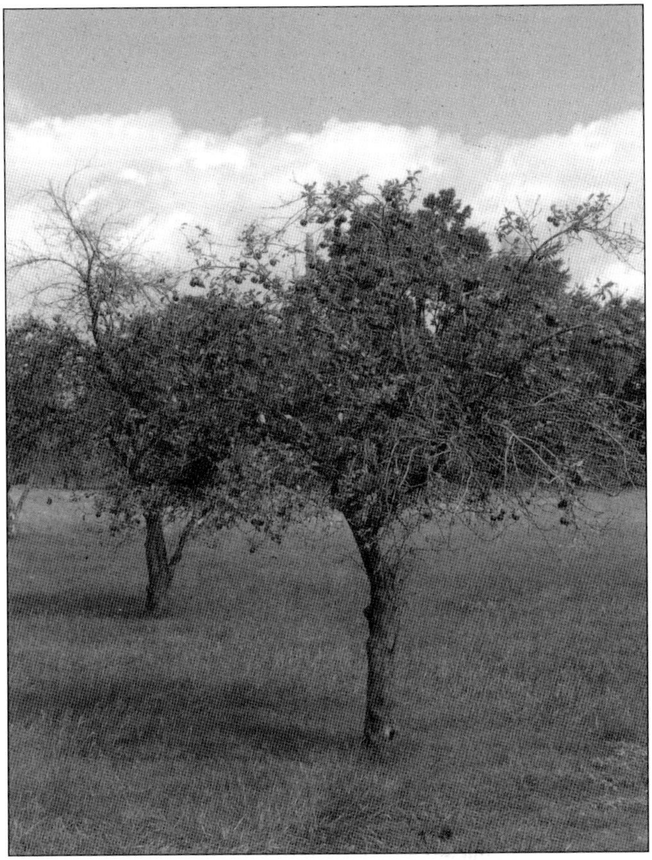

The apple orchard, located at the back of the property, was known as the "make-out" spot. Though no longer maintained or tended, the remaining trees continue to produce an annual crop. (Right, NOPH; below, photograph by author.)

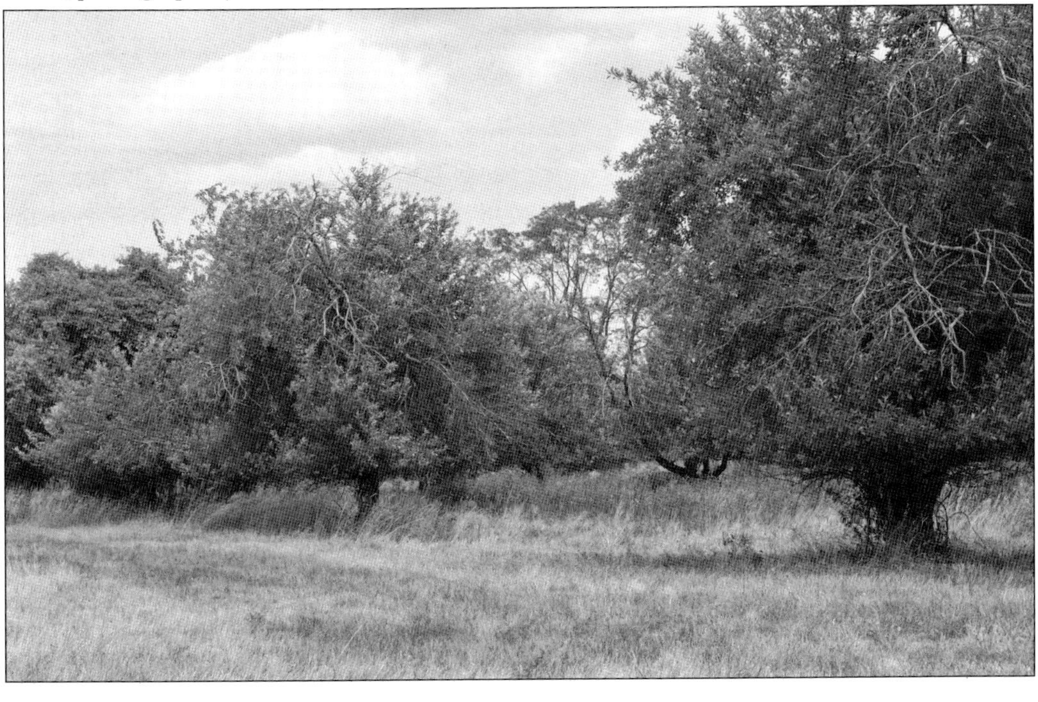

Bibliography

Art Work of Toledo, Ohio. Published in Nine Parts. Toledo, OH: Gravure Illustration Company, 1901.

Brinkerhoff, Roeliff. *Recollections of a Lifetime.* Cincinnati, OH: the Robert Clarke Company, 1900.

Cox, Clyde. *History of Toledo State Hospital.* Self-published, 1964.

Dix, Dorothea L. *Memorial to the Legislature of Massachusetts.* Boston, MA: Munroe & Francis, 1843.

Durant, Samuel W. *An Illustrated Historical Atlas of Lucas and Part of Wood Counties, Ohio.* Chicago, IL: Andreas & Baskin, 1875.

Hartung, Walter H. *History of Medical Practice in Toledo and the Maumee Valley Area, 1600–1990.* N.p., 1992.

Ohio Department of Finance. *Ohio Capital Inventory.* Columbus, OH: Department of Finance, 1962.

Van Tassel, C.S. *Men of Northwestern Ohio. A Collection of Portraits and biographies of Well Known Men in this Section of the Professional, Business, and Commercial World.* N.p., 1898.

ABOUT THE ORGANIZATION

TOLEDO STATE HOSPITAL CEMETERY RECLAMATION PROJECT

The Toledo State Hospital Cemetery Reclamation Project Committee formed in 2005, with the first members having little knowledge of the two hospital cemeteries. Interest in supporting restoration and recording the hospital's history soon brought together other volunteers from many backgrounds to begin research, promote special projects, and educate the public. Volunteers have since located and raised over 1,200 sunken burial markers, identified 80 veterans, and reconnected over 40 families with lost loved ones. Several granite memorials and a pathway beautify one cemetery, and Ohio Historical Society markers in both locations give a brief history of the hospital and the people buried there. Oral histories are collected from those having information about hospital history. Committee volunteers also oversee the collection of artifacts in the hospital's Archive Room Museum. Committee members are also available as public speakers to share hospital history with interested groups and organizations.

—Jane Graham Weber, chairperson